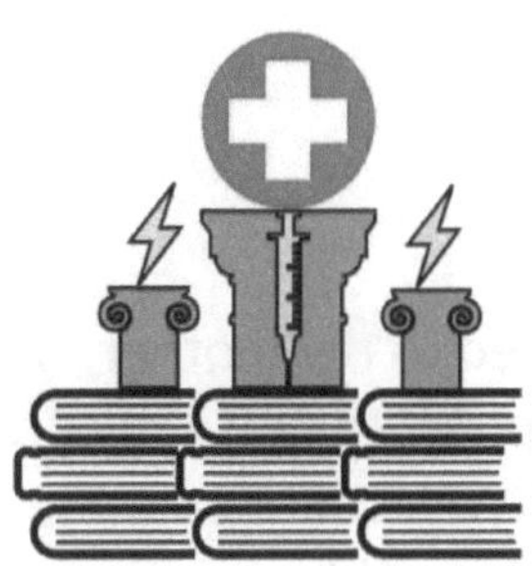

Essential Endocrine Revision for Medical Students, Residents and other Healthcare Professionals

Elite Medical Revision

Volume I: Adrenal Glands; Thyroid Gland; and Pituitary Gland & Hypothalamus

Dr. Maxim John Levy Barnett

1st Edition: 2021

Please Note: The information provided is for education and revision purposes, and should not be used as a reference for clinical decision-making. Always consult local (and national) guidelines.

Any feedback – please e-mail elitemedicalrevision@gmail.com

This book is dedicated to my mother, Dr. Deborah Levy, for her unwavering support to make my dream of becoming a doctor my reality. Without you, the creation of this revision book would not have been possible.

Contents

Yet Another Textbook (...Sigh...)

Yet another textbook (sigh)! I remember in England as a medical student maxing out my debit card on amazon towards textbooks that would serve as table coasters and TV stands, in addition to collecting dust. So why have I decided to add to the world of medical literature knowing textbooks are falling out of fashion? Three simple words: **Lectures Are Useless**! Quoting Sir William Osler (1849-1919) "...Medicine is learned by the bedside and not in the classroom...". This book has therefore been created as a 'steppingstone', to contextualise knowledge in preparation for endocrinology rotations in the upper years of medical school. Ranging from factual-based questions to case studies, this revision book provides an integrated overview in the important concepts you are likely to be expected to know and be familiar with but have never been taught (we have all been there!). This book is furthermore applicable to those wishing to simply gain a better understanding of endocrinology (the best subject in medicine) or those preparing for the United States Medical Licensing Exam (USMLE). Some of the questions are intentionally difficult, in order to reinforce likely new concepts (rather than stating 'random facts' throughout the book). By repetition in different contexts, such as lectures, ward rounds, textbooks and tests, the information will consolidate.

By picking up this book and updating your knowledge in the field of endocrinology, you already one-step ahead of those around you simply wishing to 'pass'. Whilst understanding the basics are important, one should continually aspire to improve their knowledge base (medicine is not a static subject).

Adrenal Glands

#1. A 32-year-old female with an unremarkable past medical history presents to her general practitioner with the complaint of recurrent headaches. She had originally attributed this to her last menstrual cycle (two weeks ago); however, it has recurred since. There is no pattern, with the headaches appearing at random throughout the day; during these episodes she notes a very fast heartbeat and persistent sweating. Which of the following syndromes is most associated with a phaeochromocytoma?

     a)   Neurofibromatosis Type II
     b)   Multiple Endocrine Neoplasia Type I
     c)   von-Hippel-Lindau Syndrome
     d)   Peutz-Jeghers Syndrome
     e)   von-Gierke's Disease

#2. Which of the following laboratory tests is the most appropriate initial investigation for a suspected phaeochromocytoma?

     a)   Urinary vanillylmandelic acid
     b)   Urinary dopamine
     c)   Plasma catecholamines
     d)   Urinary fractionated metanephrines
     e)   Blood Pressure and Electrocardiogram

#3. Which of the following infections is not a cause of hypoadrenalism?

     a)   Tuberculosis
     b)   Cytomegalovirus
     c)   Neisseria Meningitides
     d)   Histoplasmosis
     e)   Schistosomiasis

#4. In which of the following clinical conditions would the replacement of mineralocorticoids not be required?

     a)   Addison's Disease
     b)   Bilateral Adrenalectomy
     c)   Waterhouse-Friderichsen Syndrome
     d)   Hypophysectomy (removal of pituitary gland)
     e)   X-Linked Adrenoleukodystrophy

<u>#5.</u> A 39-year-old gentleman presents for a follow-up appointment for monitoring of his high blood pressure. His medical records reveal that despite compliance with Doxazosin, Furosemide and Atenolol, his blood pressure remains elevated at 152/96mmHg. After abstaining from his medications for two weeks, the following investigations are performed:

Aldosterone-Renin Ratio	> 30ng/dL (elevated)
Sodium	149mmol/L (135-145mmol/L)
Potassium	4.6mmol/L (3.5-5.3mmol/L)
eGFR	> 90 (normal)

Which of the following is the most likely diagnosis?
- a) Phaeochromocytoma
- b) Cushing's Syndrome
- c) Renal Artery Stenosis
- d) Conn's Syndrome
- e) Chronic Kidney Disease

<u>#6.</u> An infant is born to a newlywed Ashkenazic Jewish Couple. At birth, there is marked clitoromegaly, with the infant demonstrating lethargy. A neonatal screening test demonstrated elevated 17-hydroxyprogesterone in addition to hyponatraemia, hyperkalaemia and hypotension. What is the most likely diagnosis?
- a) Classic Congenital Adrenal Hyperplasia
- b) Non-Classic Congenital Adrenal Hyperplasia
- c) 11-Beta-Hydroxylase Deficiency
- d) 17-Alpha-Hydroxylase Deficiency
- e) Addison's Disease

<u>#7.</u> Which of the following medications must always be administered prior to levothyroxine?
- a) Labetalol
- b) Iodine
- c) Hydrocortisone
- d) 0.9% Normal Saline
- e) There is no mandated order of administration

<u>#8.</u> A mother is bathing her one-year-old son in the bathtub when she notes an abdominal 'bulge'. Concerned, she brings her son straight to the general practitioner, who performs a thorough assessment. The mass is painless, crosses the midline, and appears calcified on imaging. Moreover, the child does not display hypertension nor haematuria. On

further history taking the mother notes that the eyes seem to 'bulge' out of the socket, which she has been concerned about. Which of the following is the most likely diagnosis?

    a) Wilm's Tumour (Nephroblastoma)
    b) Neuroblastoma
    c) Phaeochromocytoma
    d) Grave's Disease
    e) Normal Child Development

#9. A 22-year-old female with a background history of well-controlled Hashimoto's Thyroiditis presents to the emergency department with vomiting, abdominal discomfort and severe dehydration. Further history taking from her boyfriend suggests that over the past three months she has begun to lose weight and become lethargic, and as a result had to drop out of her programme at the local university. Physical examination demonstrates mucosal pigmentation. Which of the following is the most important initial step of management?

    a) 100mg Hydrocortisone (Intravenous)
    b) 100mg Hydrocortisone (Oral)
    c) 100mg Fludrocortisone (Intravenous)
    d) 0.9% Normal Saline and 5% Dextrose
    e) 1.6micrograms/kilogram Levothyroxine

#10. A 23-year-old female notes a peculiar, fixed mass on her left neck, which she describes as painless. She has not noted any weight loss or fevers and is "not worried since my father and grandfather both had painless lumps in their necks without any complications". Assuming this is a paraganglioma, which mutation is most likely?

    a) Succinate Dehydrogenase Subunit D (SDHD)
    b) Succinate Dehydrogenase Subunit B (SDHB)
    c) Fumarate Dehydratase
    d) Hypoxia-Inducible Factor-1a
    e) RET Proto-oncogene

#11. Vitamins and Minerals are essential substances which fuel the metabolic pathways and are vital to normal human physiology. Which of the following deficiencies has been associated with adrenal insufficiency?

    a) Vitamin A
    b) Vitamin B12
    c) Vitamin B5

d) Magnesium
e) Selenium

<u>#12.</u> A 74-year-old male undergoes a CT of the abdomen due to a six-month history of intermittent, diffuse abdominal pain. He denies fever, weight loss or any other symptoms. A CT scan is ordered, for which a small, 1.2cm lesion is identified upon the right adrenal gland. There is no prior history of malignancy. Which of the following imaging characteristics is suggestive of a benign (incidentaloma) over a cancerous lesion?

a) Non-contrast CT attenuation below 10 Hounsefield Units
b) Non-contrast CT attenuation above 10 Hounsefield Units
c) CT washout less than 60% at 15 minutes
d) Normal 'in-phase' and 'out-of-phase' MRI Chemical Shift
e) a), c) and d)

<u>#13.</u> The adrenal gland is an endocrine organ with a unique embryological origin. The adrenal 'medulla' and 'cortex' are each derived from separate embryological tissues and display different functions. Which of the following options correctly identifies the embryological tissues of origin for both the 'medulla' and 'cortex', respectively?

a) Endoderm; Mesoderm
b) Mesoderm; Ectoderm (Neural Crest)
c) Mesoderm; Mesoderm
d) Mesoderm; Endoderm
e) Ectoderm (Neural Crest); Mesoderm

<u>#14.</u> The adrenal cortex, specifically the Zona Fasciculata, comprises the largest portion of the Adrenal Gland. The function of this layer is to produce the stress hormone, known as Cortisol. Which of the following options is the most basic precursor to the production of all steroid hormones?

a) Pregnenolone
b) 17-hydroxyprogesterone
c) Cholecalciferol
d) Cholesterol
e) Progestin

8

#15. An astute medical student is preparing his notes for the following day's lecture, for which the professor will discuss the anatomy of the adrenal glands. Anatomically, which of the following correctly describes the venous drainage of the adrenal glands?

a) The left adrenal vein drains into the left gonadal vein
b) The right adrenal vein drains into the right renal vein
c) The left adrenal vein drains into the inferior vena cava
d) The left adrenal vein drains into the left renal vein
e) The right adrenal vein drains into the left gonadal vein

#16. Which of the following corticosteroids demonstrates **no** mineralocorticoid activity?

a) Hydrocortisone
b) Prednisolone
c) Prednisone
d) Dexamethasone
e) Cortisone

#17. Which of the following best describes the term 'Adrenarche'?

a) The onset of puberty
b) The development of the adrenal gland in utero
c) The maturation of the Zona Reticularis
d) Does not occur in the presence of hypogonadism
e) A process only occurring in females

#18. SAME' (Syndrome of Apparent Mineralocorticoid Excess) is an autosomal recessive disorder characterised by a deficiency of the enzyme 11-Beta-hydroxysteroid Dehydrogenase Type II; the sequelae of this disorder include hypertension, hypernatraemia, hypokalaemia and hypoaldosteronism. Which of the following correctly identifies the function of the enzyme 11-Beta-hydroxysteroid Dehydrogenase Type II?

a) Activates Cortisone to Cortisol
b) Suppresses the release of Aldosterone
c) Increases levels of Angiotensin II
d) Inactivates Cortisol to Cortisone
e) Rate-limiting step of cortisol synthesis

#19. A 19-year-old patient receiving long-term oral prednisone for inflammatory bowel disease is being followed up for consideration to wean off of the steroids. The patient feels very well and has not noted any bleeding in her stools for well over six months (when she initiated the medication). In addition, her vital signs are normal. Her medication list includes prednisone, sulfasalazine and metronidazole. As a precaution, the general practitioner orders a full-blood count, urea & electrolytes and a C-reactive protein level. The patient is puzzled to learn that despite the absence of fever or chills, she has a WCC of 14×10^6/L (Reference: $4\text{-}9\times10^6$/L). The elevated levels of white blood cells in this patient are best exemplified as a result of:

- a) An underlying infection
- b) Haematological malignancy
- c) Laboratory error
- d) Inflammatory bowel disease flare-up
- e) Expected consequence of the medication

#20. 'Renal Tubular Acidosis' (RTA) is a disorder characterised by normal anion-gap acidosis in the setting of acidosis. Type IV RTA is the most common form, characterised by hyporeninaemic-hypoaldosteronism with hyperkalaemia. Which of the following is a common cause of this condition?

- a) Diabetes mellitus
- b) Hypertension
- c) Mercury poisoning
- d) Beta-blockers
- e) Thiazide Diuretics

#21. Prior to an elective adrenalectomy in patients with a Phaeochromocytoma, which of the following must be performed?

- a) Administration of bisoprolol, followed by phenoxybenzamine
- b) Biopsy
- c) Overnight dexamethasone suppression test
- d) Administration of bisoprolol only
- e) Administration of phenoxybenzamine, followed by bisoprolol

#22. A 24-year-old male has a background history of Addison's disease and demonstrates poor compliance with his three-times-daily regimen of hydrocortisone. His physician is planning to convert his thrice-daily regimen to once-daily prednisone. Which of the following dosages of prednisone is equivalent to 20mg of Hydrocortisone?

    a)   4mg
    b)   6mg
    c)   1/20mg
    d)   5mg
    e)   20mg

#23. An endocrinologist is currently investigating a patient with a peculiar constellation of clinical conditions. The physician notes a female of 16 years of age with Primary Adrenal Insufficiency, Type 1 Diabetes Mellitus and Hashimoto's Thyroiditis. Which of the following diagnoses is the physician likely to consider?

    a)   Autoimmune Polyglandular Syndrome Type 1
    b)   POEMS Syndrome
    c)   No genetic condition: autoimmune disorders are known to occur in clusters
    d)   Autoimmune Polyglandular Syndrome Type 2
    e)   IPEX Syndrome

#24. Cushing's Syndrome, a disorder characterised by hypercortisolism and the resultant sequelae (moon facies, truncal obesity, plethora, osteoporosis, hypertension and diabetes), is most commonly caused by:

    a)   Pituitary Tumours
    b)   Hypothalamic Tumours
    c)   Adrenal Adenomas
    d)   Medication (Iatrogenic)
    e)   Adrenal Carcinomas

#25. A 37-year-old gentleman is followed up with his Endocrinologist after resection for a medullary carcinoma of the thyroid gland. As per local guidelines, the calcitonin is measured annually, for which no abnormalities are demonstrated. The gentleman was adopted at a young age and is unaware of his family history. On physical examination the physician notes a very slender, tall male with an arm span greater than his height. This gentleman is predisposed to acquiring which of the following?

a) Phaeochromocytoma
b) Marfan's Syndrome
c) Primary Hyperparathyroidism
d) Pituitary Adenoma

#26. A 36-year-old female and her partner of 10 years have recently eloped. They would like to begin a family of their own, however, have come to the appointment due to concerns over the safety of pregnancy for the wife, who has a five-year history of Addison's Disease controlled by fludrocortisone and hydrocortisone. The advice best suited for the couple is to:
a) Avoid pregnancy, consider alternative measures
b) Discontinue fludrocortisone, continue hydrocortisone
c) Discontinue hydrocortisone, continue fludrocortisone
d) Continue both medications, however, dosage adjustments are required
e) Continue fludrocortisone, replace hydrocortisone with dexamethasone

#27. A recent immigrant to New York from Australia presents to her family physician for a checkup as part of her employment. Despite emigrating from Australia 12 months prior (and no recent travelling), the physician notes she appears rather tanned. She has a past medical history of bilateral adrenalectomy for Cushing's syndrome (unidentified source). She has since been maintained on replacement hydrocortisone and fludrocortisone without any problems. In addition to her tanned appearance, her systems review is unremarkable except for frequent headaches, which she attributes to the stress of her job in Wall Street. Which of the following options correctly identifies the likely diagnosis?
a) Addison's Disease
b) Tension-Type Headaches
c) Nelson's Syndrome
d) Haemochromatosis
e) Post-inflammatory Hyperpigmentation Syndrome

#28. Primary Aldosteronism, classically caused by an adenoma (Conn's Syndrome) is characterised by an increased serum Aldosterone-Renin Ratio (increased aldosterone, decreased renin). Prior to undergoing

this investigation, patients must withdraw which of the following medications to prevent a false-positive?
a) Doxazosin
b) Bisoprolol
c) Furosemide
d) Hydrocortisone
e) Dexamethasone

#29. Adrenal 'Incidentalomas' are lesions identified on imaging which has been requested for a separate reason. Despite their commonality, physicians must appropriately rule out malignancy and hypersecretion. Assuming a discovered 'incidentalomas' is functional (hypersecretion of a hormone), which of the following conditions is most likely to be displayed?
a) Conn's Syndrome
b) Phaeochromocytoma
c) Virilisation
d) Subclinical Cushing's Syndrome
e) Syndrome of Inappropriate Antidiuretic Hormone (SIADH) Release

#30. Which of the following is the most appropriate investigation to perform in question #29 to rule out subclinical Cushing's syndrome in an adrenal 'incidentaloma'?
a) Urinary Free Cortisol
b) Overnight Dexamethasone Suppression Test
c) Random Plasma cortisol and ACTH
d) Dexamethasone Suppression Test (8mg)
e) Levels are not measured when 'subclinical' as results will return normal

#31. Testicular Adrenal Rest Tumours ('TARTs') are commonly associated with which of the following conditions?
a) 17-alpha-hydroxylase deficiency
b) Non-classic congenital adrenal hyperplasia
c) Classic congenital adrenal hyperplasia
d) Iatrogenic Cushing's syndrome
e) Conn's Syndrome

#32. Although an extremely uncommon condition in pregnancy, gravid females in whom hypertension appears in the supine position must be considered for which endocrinological disorder?

     a) Cushing's Syndrome
     b) Addison's Disease
     c) Acromegaly
     d) Phaeochromocytoma
     e) Grave's Disease

#33. A 28-year-old male engineering student with known HIV and non-adherence to his anti-retroviral is diagnosed with a severe, fulminating fungal infection. Which of the following medications is known to inhibit cortisol synthesis within the adrenal gland?

     a) Ketoconazole
     b) Itraconazole
     c) Capsofungin
     d) Terbinafine
     e) Mifepristone

#34. Which of the following (in excess) will present akin to Syndrome of Mineralocorticoid Excess (SAME)?

     a) Tobacco
     b) Naphthylamine
     c) Liquorice
     d) Carbenoxolone
     e) a), c) and d)

#35. A third-year medical student has requested a tutorial to review Primary Aldosteronism. You explain to the student the two commonest causes are Conn's Syndrome, and Bilateral Adrenal Hyperplasia, the latter of which is the commonest. Although not used in practice, which of the following tests can be used to differentiate between Conn's Syndrome and Bilateral Adrenal Hyperplasia?

     a) Postural Test
     b) Sitting and Standing Blood Pressure
     c) 24-hour Urinary Aldosterone levels
     d) Serum Potassium Levels

#36. A 20-year-old male presents with hypertension, for which has been unresponsive to furosemide, doxazosin and atenolol. His family history is remarkable for severe hypertension (and stroke) in his mother, sister, brother and maternal grandfather. The physician is concerned the patient demonstrates Familial Hyperaldosteronism (Type I); the patient and family subsequently test positive with genetic screening. Which of the following options is the proposed treatment for the condition?

a) Angiotensin-Converting-Enzyme Inhibitors
b) Glucocorticoids
c) Spironolactone
d) Thiazide Diuretics
e) Adrenalectomy

#37. A 56-year-old gentleman is subsequently diagnosed with Conn's after the discovery of an adrenal 'incidentaloma'. The patient adamantly refuses to undergo surgery for an adrenalectomy, as his wife underwent general anaesthesia for a hysterectomy and 'never woke up'. It is decided that this gentleman will be treated with a mineralocorticoid receptor antagonist, Spironolactone. Which of the following side-effects must this gentleman be warned about?

a) Hypokalaemia
b) Masculinization
c) Chronic Cough
d) Gynaecomastia
e) Headache

#38. After developing the side-effect listed in question #37, returns for a follow-up appointment three months later and has discontinued all blood pressure medications (against medical advice). His most recent blood results demonstrate the following:

Sodium	150mmol/L (135-145mmol/L)
Potassium	3.2mmol/L (3.5-5.3mmol/L)
eGFR	> 90 (normal)

This gentleman has been complaining of increased urination, dehydration and muscular weakness. Which of the following is the most likely cause of the presenting symptom?

a) Hypertension has caused renal damage
b) Hypernatraemia-induced nephrogenic diabetes insipidus
c) Hypokalaemia-induced nephrogenic diabetes insipidus
d) Hypokalaemia-induced central diabetes insipidus
e) Hypernatraemia-induced central diabetes insipidus

#39. Phaeochromocytomas are predominantly hyper-functioning, whereas paraganglioma may be either silent (parasympathetic) or hyper-functioning (sympathetic). Which of the following hormones is solely produced within the adrenal gland (its presence may imply a phaeochromocytoma)?

    a) Dopamine
    b) Normetanephrine
    c) Metanephrine
    d) Epinephrine
    e) Norepinephrine

#40. A recently wed couple, who are both known carriers of 21-alpha-hydroxylase deficiency, would like to start a family. The mother asks if there is any medication, she can take during pregnancy to prevent 'virilisation' of the foetus. Although still considered experimental, the following medication may be taken under guidance of a consultant to prevent virilisation of a female foetus:

    a) Triamcinolone
    b) Spironolactone
    c) Diethylstilbestrol
    d) Hydrocortisone
    e) Dexamethasone

#41. A class of medical students are being taught how to prescribe corticosteroids. Following the natural circadian rhythm of cortisol release, when at what time of the day should the highest dosage (of a three-times-per-day regimen) of a corticosteroid be administered?

    a) Lunchtime
    b) Two hours after lunch
    c) Bedtime
    d) Morning
    e) Two hours before dinner

#42. An elderly gentleman is being investigated for a three-month history of weight loss, unexplained fevers and cachexia. He has noted an occasional cough over the past five months, however stopped smoking one year ago (previously, 30-pack-year history). Physical examination is notable for clubbing. A CT scan of the chest-abdomen-pelvis demonstrates an enlarged, 6x3cm irregular mass on his right adrenal gland. The location of the primary malignancy is most likely which of the following organs?

a) Melanocytes
b) Prostate
c) Proximal Convoluted Tubule
d) Lungs
e) Liver

#43. Understanding the anatomy of the adrenal gland is of vital importance when performing a surgical operation on the adrenal gland or renal tissue. Which of the following layers of fat separates the adrenal glands from the kidneys?

a) Perirenal
b) Pararenal
c) Periadrenal
d) Reno-Adrenal
e) None of the above

#44. The adrenal cortex and adrenal medulla, although are derived from distinct embryological tissues, develop concurrently. Around which week of gestation do the adrenal cortex and medulla begin to develop?

a) 2-3 weeks
b) 5-6 weeks
c) 9-10 weeks
d) 12-14 weeks
e) 15-16 weeks

#45. The adrenal cortex is divided into three layers (zona glomerulosa, zona fasciculata and zona reticularis). Within the developing foetus, however, the adrenal cortex is divided into two main zones, with a predominant function to release sex hormones. Premature infants may therefore display a 'transient' state of adrenal insufficiency as the 'switch' to producing cortisol and aldosterone has not yet occurred. Which of the following correctly lists the two predominant zones of the foetal adrenal cortex?

a) Glomerular Zone; Foetal Zone
b) Foetal Zone; Definitive Zone
c) Definitive Zone; Glomerular Zone
d) Reticular Zone; Definitive Zone
e) Foetal Zone; Reticular Zone

#46. A rather infrequent disorder is characterised by the colloquial term 'Triple A Syndrome'. This is distinct from an abdominal aortic aneurysm, and refers to the constellation of ACTH Resistance, Absent Lacrimation and which of the following options?

    a) Aortic Insufficiency
    b) Achalasia
    c) Aortic Aneurysm
    d) Atrophic Gastritis
    e) Atrial Fibrillation

#47. A 17-year-old boy is brought to the family physician by his parents, who are very concerned with his behaviour. He is repeating grade 11 as he became very hyperactive and disruptive at school over the past year. The parents note this was quite a strange occurrence, as he has always been well behaved prior to this past year. Despite once being the top student and achieving honour roll, he no longer focuses and has stopped turning in assignments. He has been complaining of severe headaches, muscle stiffness and difficulty initiating urination. He reluctantly admits that he no longer is able to achieve an erection and his girlfriend has broken up with him. He denies any illicit usage of drugs and demonstrates a positive mood and affect. In the last week, he has begun to feel nauseous upon awakening, and very weak. When standing up after sitting in a chair at school, he has fallen over and vomited on multiple occasions, requiring him to be sent home and miss the rest of the school day. His mother is very concerned, as her brother demonstrated a similar presentation in his early 20's, but never received medical care and passed away quite soon thereafter. Which of the following correctly identifies the diagnosis, and an available medication?

    a) Wilson's Disease; Penicillamine
    b) Krabbe's Disease; no treatment
    c) Tay-Sachs Disease; no treatment
    d) X-Linked Adrenoleukodystrophy; Lorenzo's Oil
    e) Fabry's Disease; Recombinant alpha-galactosidase A

#48. An obese 9-year-old patient is followed-up by the paediatric team. He has a known history of recurrent hyperphagia, for which medication and psychological intervention have proved unhelpful. His stature is below the tenth centile for his gender and age, and he furthermore is noted to suffer with intellectual disability. After a full physical examination, he is noted to demonstrate a micro-penis. The paediatric team consider a genetic cause for this presentation, and perform a genetic test, which reveals uniparental maternal disomy of chromosome 15. Which of the following options correctly lists the diagnosis, and a potential endocrine complication?

> a) Noonan Syndrome; Adrenal Incidentaloma
> b) Mosaic Turner Syndrome; ectopic ACTH Syndrome
> c) Prader-Willi Syndrome; Central Adrenal Insufficiency
> d) Noonan Syndrome; Primary Adrenal Insufficiency
> e) Prader-Willi Syndrome; Primary Adrenal Insufficiency

#49. The release of aldosterone can be inhibited by which of the following?

> a) Atrial Natriuretic Peptide
> b) Angiotensin II
> c) Dopamine
> d) a) and b)
> e) a) and c)

#50. The rate-limiting step for the synthesis of catecholamines is for which of the following enzymes?

> a) DOPA Decarboxylase
> b) Tyrosine Hydroxylase
> c) Dopamine Beta Hydroxylase
> d) Phenylalanine Hydroxylase
> e) Phenylethanolamine N-Methyltransferase

#51. von-Hippel Lindau may be subdivided into multiple categories; which of the following subtypes encompasses Phaeochromocytoma, CNS Haemangioblastoma and Renal Cell Carcinoma?

> a) Type 1
> b) Type 2A
> c) Type 2B
> d) Type 2C
> e) Type 3

#52. All of the following are associated with increased serum aldosterone levels except for:

> a) Type IV Renal Tubular Acidosis
> b) Spironolactone

c) Gordon's Syndrome
d) Liddle's Syndrome
e) a) and d)

#53. Which of the following options is a validated histological scoring system which can be used to determine if an adrenal incidentaloma is likely benign or malignant?
a) Weiss Criteria
b) PASS Criteria
c) GAPP Criteria
d) Burch and Wartofsky Criteria
e) None of the above

#54. All of the following are potential complications of a biopsy from an adrenal incidentaloma in a 72-year-old gentleman with an unremarkable medical history, except for:
a) Pneumothorax
b) Haemorrhage
c) Pancreatitis
d) Tumour Seeding
e) Catecholaminergic Crisis
f) Adrenal Insufficiency

#55. Adrenal biopsies are typically not advocated for in the presence of an adrenal incidentaloma due to the myriad of potential complications. Which of the following options is correct regarding a biopsy for an adrenal incidentaloma?
a) Cannot distinguish carcinoma from adenoma
b) May distinguish carcinoma from adenoma
c) Failure rate of 90%
d) Cannot detect if malignancy is of extra-adrenal source
e) None of the above

#56. Which of the following terms correctly defines the clinical finding of two histologically distinct (albeit adjacent) neoplasms within the adrenal gland?
a) Bisequential Malignancy
b) Collision tumour
c) Multi-histological neoplasm
d) None of the above

#57. A 62-year-old female is referred to the endocrine department by her general practitioner due to the complain of overwhelming anxiety, palpitations, sweating and sense of impending doom. These 'anxiety' attacks occur at random, and as far as the patient is aware, they are not triggered by anything. There is no family history of note. Which of the following medications must be withheld prior to investigating for a phaeochromocytoma, or will lead to elevated urinary catecholamine levels?

    a) Amitriptyline
    b) Clonidine
    c) Guanethidine
    d) Tranylcypromine
    e) All of the above must be withheld

#58. Very long chain fatty acids may accumulate and lead to adrenal insufficiency in which of the following clinical disorders?

    a) Zellweger Syndrome
    b) X-Linked Adrenoleukodystrophy
    c) IMAGe Syndrome
    d) Metachromatic Leukodystrophy
    e) Hunter's Syndrome

#59. Adrenal insufficiency with autoantibodies directed towards Interferon-Omega is suggestive for which of the following disorders?

    a) Autoimmune Polyglandular Syndrome Type 1
    b) Addison's Disease
    c) Autoimmune Polyglandular Syndrome Type 3
    d) Liddle's Syndrome
    e) None of the above

#60. Despite optimal replacement with corticosteroids and mineralocorticoids in primary adrenal insufficiency, many females continue to demonstrate an impaired quality of life (including fatigue, impaired concentration, decreased bone mineral density, altered libido and diminished axillary hair). Which of the following may be trialled for six months in female patients with adrenal insufficiency?

    a) Dehydroepiandrosterone 25-50mg
    b) Testosterone 1mg oral gel
    c) Dehydroepiandrosterone-sulphate 25-50mg
    d) a) and c)
    e) None of the above

#61. A 32-year-old husband and 31-year-old female present to the endocrine clinic. They would like to begin a family; however, they are concerned as they are known carriers for congenital adrenal hyperplasia. They would like to know what is the likelihood they will give birth to a child who will be healthy (neither a carrier, nor affected)?

a) 75%
b) 50%
c) 25%
d) Male: 50%; Female: 25%
e) Not enough information

#62. The non-classic form of congenital adrenal hyperplasia is rather confusingly more common than the classic form. It often presents in early adulthood and can be confirmed with a synacthen stimulation test demonstrating elevated 17-hydroxyprogesterone. In a 29-year-old male engineering student with incidentally discovered non-classic congenital adrenal hyperplasia, which of the following is the most appropriate treatment regimen?

a) Lifelong mineralocorticoid replacement
b) Lifelong Androgen Receptor Antagonist therapy
c) Lifelong glucocorticoid replacement
d) Six-month trial of glucocorticoid and mineralocorticoid replacement
e) No treatment is recommended

#63. All of the following may alter the results of a urinary free cortisol measurement except for:

a) Combined Oral Contraceptive Pills
b) Renal Failure
c) Obesity
d) Excessive intake of water

#64. A 1mg overnight dexamethasone suppression test is appropriate for which of the following situations when screening for Cushing's Syndrome?

a) Nephrotic Syndrome
b) Renal Failure
c) Incidentaloma
d) a) and b)
e) b) and c)

<u>#65.</u> A final-year-medical student is sitting in with the local endocrine consultant in his clinic. The consultant presents to the student a CT of the abdomen with a confirmed adrenal incidentaloma. The consultant then goes on to explain that the patient demonstrated an abnormal dexamethasone suppression test, in addition to low ACTH levels. The consultant then asks the medical student what he thinks the likely diagnosis is, to which the student responds he is unsure if this is Cushing's Disease or Cushing's Syndrome. Which of the following is the correct response?

a)   Cushing's Disease refers to an adrenal mass, whereas Cushing's Syndrome is an umbrella term for any cause of Cushing's
b)   Cushing's Disease and Cushing's Syndrome are interchangeable
c)   Cushing's Syndrome refers to an adrenal mass, whereas Cushing's Disease is an umbrella term for any cause of Cushing's
d)   Cushing's Disease refers to a pituitary mass, whereas Cushing's Syndrome is an umbrella term for any cause of Cushing's
e)   Cushing's Syndrome refers to a pituitary mass, whereas Cushing's Disease is an umbrella term for any cause of Cushing's

<u>#66.</u> Which of the following conditions will present with high-renin, high-aldosterone and normotension?

a)   Reninoma
b)   Renal artery stenosis
c)   Bartter's Syndrome
d)   Liddle's Syndrome
e)   c) and d)

<u>#67.</u> A 74-year-old gentleman is noted to have non-specific abdominal discomfort. He denies any systemic symptoms or weight loss, however, the junior doctors decide to order a CT scan of the abdomen, for which a resultant 2.3cm adrenal adenoma is discovered. He is noted to demonstrate hypertension whilst staying in hospital (154/94mmHg). The following results are obtained:

Plasma Renin [UPRIGHT]	9pmol/L/hour (Ref: 2.8-4.5)
Plasma Aldosterone [UPRIGHT]	700pmol/L (Ref: 100-800)
eGFR	> 90 (normal)

Low-Dose 1mg Overnight Dexamethasone Suppression Test	8AM Cortisol 49nmol/L (Ref: <55nmol/L)
24 Hour Urine Free Normetadrenaline	2.4micromol/day (Ref: 0-3)
24-Hour Urine Free Metadrenaline	1.2micromol/day (Ref: 0-1.8)

What is the most likely diagnosis?

- a) Conn's Syndrome
- b) Phaeochromocytoma
- c) Bilateral Adrenal Hyperplasia
- d) Adrenocortical Carcinoma
- e) Incidentaloma and concurrent essential hypertension

#68. A 22-year-old gentleman attends a follow-up appointment at the endocrinology department. This gentleman is displaying hypertension and poor glycaemic control, despite a healthy diet and daily exercise. He denies any illicit substance abuse and does not take any regular medications (prescribed or over the counter). He is unaware of his family history as he was adopted at a young age. The physician performs a physical examination, which notes thinning of the dermis, easy bruising and various pigmented lesions over his skin. Moreover, he notes the patient demonstrates difficulty arising from a seated position when asked to transfer to the examination bed. A cardiovascular examination is prominent for a murmur over the left precordium, with a characteristic 'plop' sound. The physician requests the following investigations:

24 Hour Urinary Free Cortisol	Greater than 4x upper limit of normal (elevated)
Low-dose dexamethasone test	Cortisol remains elevated
ACTH	Undetectable
eGFR	> 90mL/min/1.73m^2 (normal)
Fasting Plasma Glucose	11.2mmol/L
CT Abdomen	Multiple (Bilateral) Adrenal Nodules Identified

What is the most likely diagnosis?

- a) Cushing's Disease
- b) Primary Pigmented Nodular Adrenocortical Disease (PPNAD)
- c) Phaeochromocytoma
- d) The Carney Complex
- e) b) and d)

#69. With reference to question #68, what is the most likely explanation for the 'plop' identified on auscultation?

- a) Mitral Valve Prolapse

b) Aortic Insufficiency
c) Cardiac Myxoma
d) Cardiac Rhabdomyosarcoma
e) Combined Aortic Insufficiency and Stenosis

#70. Which of the following options suggests Macronodular Adrenal Hyperplasia over Primary Pigmented Nodular Adrenocortical Disease?
a) Young age
b) Histology: Atrophic tissue between nodules
c) CT Scan: String of Beads Appearance
d) Associated with the Carney Complex
e) Associated with McCune-Albright Syndrome, Multiple Endocrine Neoplasia (Type I) and/or Familial Adenomatous Polyposis
f) Aberrant hormone expression
g) Increase in cortisol during Liddle's Test
h) e) and f)

#71. Which of the following options correctly characterises a chemodectoma?
a) Sympathetic paraganglioma
b) More common amongst males
c) More common at high-altitude
d) Hypersecretes hormones
e) Fontaine's Sign positive
f) c) and e)

#72. Apart of the adrenal medulla, which of the following is the only other organ which contains the enzyme PNMT (Phenylethanolamine N-methyltransferase)?
a) Zona Glomerulosa of Adrenal Cortex
b) Seminiferous Tubules of Testes
c) Graafian Follicle
d) Carotid Body
e) Organ of Zuckerkandl

#73. A female patient in her early 20s is evaluated in the endocrine department for follow-up after removal of a chemodectoma. Her family history is unremarkable, and genetic analysis did not identify a familial mutation. The physician notes this patient 's recent chest x-ray was reported as abnormal, due to the presence of a calcified lung nodule; further investigation demonstrated a histological confirmation of a pulmonary chondroma. If this patient were to develop a gastrointestinal stromal tumour, what would be the likely underlying diagnosis?

a) Carney-Stratakis Dyad
b) The Carney Complex
c) Tuberous Sclerosis
d) The Carney Triad
e) Familial Paraganglioma

#74. With reference to question #73, if this patient were to demonstrate a chemodectoma and gastrointestinal tumour (no pulmonary chondroma) in addition to a positive family history, which of the following would be the likely diagnosis?

a) Carney-Stratakis Dyad
b) The Carney Complex
c) Tuberous Sclerosis
d) The Carney Triad
e) Familial Paraganglioma

#75. Which of the following is a potential complication of corticosteroid administration?

a) Increase serum TSH
b) Diabetes Insipidus
c) Hypoglycaemia
d) Hyperandrogenaemia
e) b) and d)

#76. A 72-year-old gentleman with a known history of prostatic carcinoma is brought to emergency department by his wife, who noted her husband to be complaining of severe back pain and urinary incontinence. A full-spine MRI demonstrates vertebral metastases, with cord compression. An 8mg bolus of Dexamethasone is prescribed as per local guidelines. Which of the following medications must also be prescribed in this gentleman?

a) Fludrocortisone
b) Abiraterone
c) Finasteride
d) Omeprazole
e) None of the above

#77. A 34-year-old gentleman is reviewed in the endocrine clinic for a follow-up appointment after a diagnosis of adrenal insufficiency. Three months prior, he was involved in a motorcycle accident, for which he acquired traumatic brain injury with resultant hypopituitarism. He has been prescribed 25mg Hydrocortisone (10mg morning, 10mg lunch, 5 mg afternoon) and the patient wishes to discuss the merits of beginning growth hormone replacement. Which of the following is a potential effect of initiating growth hormone replacement in this patient?

a) Growth hormone will inhibit 11-Beta-Hydroxysteroid Dehydrogenase Type I, leading to hyporcortisolism at the current dose
b) Growth hormone will induce 11-Beta-Hydroxysteroid Dehydrogenase Type I, leading to hypecortisolism at the current dose
c) Growth Hormone may worsen the glycaemic status
d) a) and c)
e) b) and c)

#78. A 64-year-old women with a three-month history of weight gain and lethargy presents to her family physician. The physician notes a reddish complexion, proximal muscular atrophy and multiple bruises across her upper limbs. Five months ago, she suffered a fracture of her humeral head when lifting the groceries out of her car. Her only significant medical history is the commencement of transdermal oestrogen (hormone replacement therapy) two weeks ago for uncontrollable hot flushes. Her physician queries Cushing's syndrome. Which of the following statements is true regarding the dexamethasone suppression testing?

a) Transdermal oestrogen increases total cortisol
b) Oral oestrogen has decreases total cortisol
c) Transdermal oestrogen decreases total cortisol
d) Transdermal oestrogen has no effect upon total cortisol
e) Both oral and transdermal oestrogen must be stopped six weeks prior to a low-dose dexamethasone suppression test

#79. A medical student sitting in on the adrenal clinic is quizzed by the consultant regarding adrenal disorders. What are the two most important criteria to be assessed when an adrenal incidentaloma is identified?

a) (1) Is the mass benign or malignant; (2) What is the size of the mass?
b) (1) What is the size of the mass; (2) What is the medication History?
c) (1) Is the mass benign or malignant; (2) Is there a history of familial syndromes?
d) (1) Is the mass benign or malignant; (2) Is the mass functional or non-functional
e) (1) Is the mass benign or malignant; (2) Was the mass identified via non-contrast CT or MRI?

<u>#80.</u> The medical student is question #79 is further quizzed; around what percentage of adrenal incidentalomas are silent (non-functional)?

a) 1-10%
b) 20-40%
c) 50-60%
d) 70-90%
e) Virtually 100%

<u>#81.</u> A 65-year-old male presents to his general practitioner at the insistence of his daughter. Over the past three years the daughter has noted a distinct change in the appearance of her father. Despite reassurance from many different doctors over the past few years, this has progressed. Physical examination is remarkable for carpal tunnel syndrome, prognathism, goitre and a displaced apex beat. Which of the following conditions may lead to this disorder as a consequence of paraneoplastic syndrome?

a) Adrenal Adenoma
b) Adrenal Carcinoma
c) Conn's Syndrome
d) Phaeochromocytoma
e) Pituitary Metastases to the Adrenal Gland

<u>#82.</u> During pregnancy, in patients with primary aldosteronism, what is the natural course of the disease?

a) Hypertension worsens during pregnancy
b) Hypertension improves during pregnancy
c) Hypertension neither improves nor worsens

d)   a) or b)

#83. In a patient with addison's disease prescribed 20mg of hydrocortisone daily, which of the following is the best advice to give during a minor illness (such as a respiratory tract infection)
- a)   Seek immediate medical attention
- b)   Administer the spare 100mg Hydrocortisone IM syringe
- c)   Continue regular dosage
- d)   Administer three-times usual daily dose for three days; seek medical attention if no improvement by day four

#84. In which of the following cohorts is hypoglycaemia a more likely presentation of adrenal insufficiency?
- a)   Primary adrenal insufficiency
- b)   Adults
- c)   Secondary Adrenal Insufficiency
- d)   Children
- e)   c) and d)
- f)   a) and b)

#85. Autoantibodies directed towards which of the following compounds are present in greater than 90% of patients with addison's disease?
- a)   11-hydroxylase
- b)   21-hydroxylase
- c)   17-hydroxylase
- d)   3-beta-hydroxysteroid-dehydrogenase
- e)   Interferon-Omega

#86. In the presence of concurrent primary hypertension and primary adrenal insufficiency, which of the following is the correct management?
- a)   Avoid mineralocorticoids
- b)   Prescribe mineralocorticoids with low-dose mineralocorticoid antagonist
- c)   Increase salt intake
- d)   Decrease salt intake
- e)   a) and d)

#87. MIBG (Metaiodobenzylguanidine) is used to scan for paragangliomas/phaeochromocytomas when the CT and/or MRI does not demonstrate an intra-abdominal neoplasm (with biochemical and clinical evidence of a paraganglioma/phaeochromocytoma). Which of the following mediations may interfere with MIBG uptake and lead to a spurious result?

    a) Amitriptyline
    b) Phenoxybenzamine
    c) Ibuprofen
    d) a) and b)
    e) b) and c)

#88. Serum Aldosterone-Renin ratio is the gold-standard screening test for an aldosteronoma. In which of the following situations will this test become unreliable?

    a) eGFR below $15mL/min/1.73m^2$
    b) K^+: 3.1mmol/mol
    c) Ibuprofen administration
    d) Advanced age
    e) All of the above

#89. A 23-year-old female presents to the emergency department with an Addisonian crisis. She has a longstanding history of poor compliance to medication and recurrent admissions. She is administered 100mg of Intravenous Hydrocortisone in addition to three litres of normal saline. Over the following three days she is tapered to an oral stress dose. On day five she is noted to have difficulty swallowing her medication and complains of a headache. Soon after she is complaining of an inability to move her lower limbs. Which of the following best describes the diagnosis and causative factor?

    a) Steroid Psychosis; Hydrocortisone
    b) Cerebral Oedema; Hydrocortisone
    c) Central Pontine Myelinolysis; Hydrocortisone
    d) Central Pontine Myelinolysis; Saline
    e) Cerebral Haemorrhage; Hydrocortisone

#90. A 62-year-old male is under investigation for refractory hypertension. Despite treatment with ramipril, amlodipine and bisoprolol, his blood pressure averages 164/92mmHg. His family physician had commenced him on Bendroflumethiazide, however he developed severe, symptomatic hypokalaemia over the following weeks, and this was immediately discontinued. His potassium is corrected, and he undergoes the following investigations:

Aldosterone	1,360 pmol/L (100-800)
Plasma Renin Activity	1.6pmol/hr (2.8-4.5)
eGFR	89mL/min/1.73m^2
Saline Infusion Test (2L Normal Saline) [SEATED POSITION]	Plasma Aldosterone after four hours: 15ng/dL (<10ng/dL)

A CT abdomen reports no specific abnormalities identified. Which of the following is the next appropriate step for this patient?

    a)   MIBG
    b)   Positron-Emission-Tomography
    c)   MRI Abdomen
    d)   Selective Adrenal Venous Sampling
    e)   No further tests required; initiate mineralocorticoid receptor antagonist

#91. Neuroblastomas are most commonly found in the adrenal gland, however, may be identified throughout the sympathetic nervous system. Which of the following genes is typically amplified in a neuroblastoma?

    a)   c-myc
    b)   k-myc
    c)   n-myc
    d)   vHL
    e)   a), b) or c)

#92. 11-Beta-Hydroxylase Deficiency accounts for no more than five percent of cases of Congenital Adrenal Hyperplasia. In which of the following groups is this disease most prevalent (likely a founder effect)?

    a)   Ashkenazi Jews (German Ancestry)
    b)   Sephardic Jews (Moroccan Ancestry)
    c)   Northern Europeans
    d)   Afro-Caribbean
    e)   Indian subcontinent

#93. A male infant is noted to have an omphalocoele, large tongue and recurrent unexplained episodes of lethargy. Further evaluation suggests the left-side of his body is more developed compared to that of the left (larger). This infant is at an increased risk for both a Wilm's Tumour and which of the following adrenal disorders?

    a)   X-Linked Adrenoleukodystrophy
    b)   Addison's Disease
    c)   Phaeochromocytoma
    d)   Cushing's Syndrome
    e)   Conn's Syndrome

#94. Occasionally, the serum levels of Chromogranin A and Chromogranin B are measured when the diagnosis of a phaeochromocytoma is suspected. Which of the following may lead to an increased serum level of Chromogranin A?

    a)   Omeprazole
    b)   Eating
    c)   Heterophile Antibody Interference
    d)   Pernicious Anaemia
    e)   All of the above

#95. All of the following corticosteroids may interfere with a serum cortisol assay except for which of the following?

    a)   Triamcinolone
    b)   Hydrocortisone
    c)   Dexamethasone
    d)   Prednisolone
    e)   Prednisone

#96. During a medical school lecture, the professor explains between 10-20mg of cortisol are released each day from the adrenal cortex. He then asks the audience how much aldosterone is released from the adrenal cortex each day? Which of the following is the correct response?

    a)   10-20 mg
    b)   10-20 micrograms
    c)   100-150 mg
    d)   100-150 micrograms
    e)   1 g

#97. Conn's Syndrome, very infrequently, has been reported in which of the following familial syndromes?

    a)   Neurofibromatosis Type I
    b)   Von-Hippel-Lindau Syndrome

c) Multiple Endocrine Neoplasia Type 1
d) Neurofibromatosis Type II
e) The Carney Complex

#98. Which of the following best described the term 'adrenopause'?
a) Decline in the release of cortisol with increasing age
b) Decline in the release of aldosterone with increasing age
c) Decline in the release of dehydroepiandrosterone (DHEA) and dehydroepiandrosterone-sulfate (DHEA-s) with increasing age
d) Decline in the secretion of all hormones released from the adrenal gland with increasing age
e) None of the above

#99. A 65-year-old female with a past history of both breast cancer and leukaemia, is evaluated for sudden onset virilisation. Genetic analysis demonstrates an inactivating mutation of the p-53 tumour suppressor gene. Which of the following options correctly lists both the current condition and likely underlying clinical disorder?
a) Adrenocortical Carcinoma; Multiple Endocrine Neoplasia
b) Adrenocortical Carcinoma; von-Hippel-Lindau Syndrome
c) Adrenocortical Carcinoma; Li-Fraumeni Syndrome
d) Adrenocortical Carcinoma; BRCA1 mutation

#100. Addison's Disease may present with which of the following biochemical results?
a) Hyperglycaemia
b) Hypercalcaemia
c) Hypernatraemia
d) Hypomagnesaemia
e) Hypocalcaemia

Adrenal Glands – Answers

<u>#1</u>. c) von-Hippel-Lindau Syndrome
von-Hippel-Lindau Syndrome is characterised by renal cell carcinoma, cerebellar, spinal and retinal haemangioblastomas, phaeochromocytomas and pancreatic neuroendocrine tumours.

<u>#2.</u> d) Urinary fractionated metanephrines
Either urinary or plasma fractionated metanephrines are first-line investigations for the diagnosis of a phaeochromocytoma. Urinary fractionated metanephrines are preferred due to the higher specificity compared to plasma fractionated metanephrines.

<u>#3.</u> e) Schistosomiasis
Adrenal damage is not associated with schistosomiasis; all other options listed may lead to adrenal destruction. Tuberculosis is the most common cause of primary adrenal insufficiency within the developing world and was the original description of Addison's Disease. Cytomegalovirus is well-documented as causing adrenalitis (and eventual destruction) in the immunocompromised. Neisseria Meningitides may lead to wide-spread sepsis and resultant adrenal damage from haemorrhagic infarction, known as Waterhouse-Friderichsen Syndrome. Histoplasmosis is a fungal infection which can mimic tuberculosis in immunocompromised patients and is a well-known cause of adrenal insufficiency.

<u>#4.</u> d) Hypophysectomy
This would constitute secondary adrenal insufficiency, for which glucocorticoid replacement is mandatory (under the influence of ACTH), however, the Renin-Angiotensin-Aldosterone System is intact (therefore mineralocorticoids are unnecessary). All other options listed are causes of primary adrenal insufficiency, whereby mineralocorticoids must be replaced.

<u>#5.</u> d) Conn's Syndrome
It is important to note that up to 40% of patients with primary aldosteronism may demonstrate normokalaemia. A Phaeochromocytoma is rare and does not fit with the demonstrated blood results; his young age and refractory (rather than episodic) hypertension suggest Primary Aldosteronism. There is nothing in the

history to suggest Cushing's Syndrome, which would not present with an elevated aldosterone-renin ratio. Renal Artery Stenosis is a classic differential diagnosis of refractory hypertension; however, this would be a cause of secondary aldosteronism, with a lowered aldosterone-renin ratio, and likely presents at an older age (classically, a bruit is noted on physical examination). Chronic kidney disease is not likely as the patient demonstrates a normal eGFR.

#6. a) Classic Congenital Adrenal Hyperplasia
Congenital Adrenal Hyperplasia is prevalent amongst Ashkenazic Jewish Patients; most commonly, this is a mutation in the gene encoding for 21-alpha hydroxylase enzyme. This results in the inability to create both cortisol and aldosterone, leading to shunting towards androgen synthesis. This displays as hypotonia, hyponatraemia, hyperkalaemia, and virilisation (such as clitoromegaly). Neonatal screening tests demonstrate an elevated 17-hydroxyprogesterone.

#7. c) Hydrocortisone
Levothyroxine, if administered before hydrocortisone will increase hydrocortisone's metabolism and precipitate an Addisonian (adrenal) crisis. Therefore, hydrocortisone must be delivered prior to the administration of levothyroxine.

#8. b) Neuroblastoma
A neuroblastoma can occasionally be difficult to differentiate from a Wilm's Tumour, however, as in the case study, a neuroblastoma will cross the midline and is calcified on imaging. Neuroblastoma may metastasise to the bones and periorbital tissues (demonstrating proptosis), in addition to a 'blueberry muffin' rash and opsoclonus-myoclonus syndrome. Hypertension is less likely with a neuroblastoma.

#9. a) 100mg Hydrocortisone (Intravenous)
Patients with autoimmune thyroiditis (as well as diabetes mellitus type 1, coeliac's disease and pernicious anaemia) are at risk of developing another autoimmune condition such as Addison's Disease, which this patient is presenting with. During a crisis, a stress dosage of 100mg Hydrocortisone Intravenously is delivered - it is not appropriate to give oral medication as she is vomiting and will not absorb the dosage. Fludrocortisone is not necessary as high dosages of hydrocortisone demonstrate mineralocorticoid effects (40mg Hydrocortisone demonstrates roughly 100mg Fludrocortisone). Normal saline and

dextrose are important in the management but are not the most important and initial step. If this patient requires levothyroxine, it cannot be given before steroids as this will precipitate an adrenal crisis (by metabolising the steroids). Fludrocortisone is further not prescribed during an adrenal crisis as it takes a few days to begin to demonstrate any effect, and the sodium load within the intravenous saline will provide the sodium replacement in the interim.

#10. a) Succinate Dehydrogenase Subunit D (SDHD)
Familial Paraganglioma Syndrome (as demonstrated in this case scenario) is most commonly Type I, which involves a mutation in the Succinate Dehydrogenase (subunit D) enzyme. One should be aware that the presence of renal cell carcinoma or malignancy/metastases suggests Subunit B mutation. As with the case presentation, parasympathetic (and hence inactive) paraganglioma may develop, commonly within the head and neck region.

#11. c) Vitamin B5 (Pantothenic Acid)
A deficiency of Vitamin B5 has been associated with adrenal insufficient states.

#12. a) Non-Contrast CT attenuation below 10 Hounsefield Units
Around 70% of 'incidentalomas' of the adrenal gland are lipid-rich and therefore demonstrate an attenuation of less than 10 Hounsefield Units on a non-contrast CT. Suspicious lesions (and phaeochromocytomas) demonstrate a lipid attenuation above 10 Hounsefield Units. For comparison, water is 0 Hounsefield Units. An incidentaloma would demonstrate a washout of contrast of greater than (not less than) 60% at 15 minutes. Similarly, 'incidentalomas' would demonstrate a normal 'in-phase' MRI, but a disordered 'out-of-phase' MRI chemical shift.

#13. e) Ectoderm (Neural Crest); Mesoderm
The adrenal medulla is formed from the neural crest cells (Ectoderm derivative), with the adrenal cortex formed from the mesoderm.

#14. d) Cholesterol
Cholesterol is the precursor to all steroid hormone synthesis.

#15. d) The left adrenal vein drains into the left renal vein
The right adrenal vein drains directly into the inferior vena cava, with the left adrenal vein draining into the left renal vein. For this reason, the left adrenal vein is easier to catheterise as it is longer than the right adrenal vein (3cm versus 1cm).

#16. d) Dexamethasone
Dexamethasone demonstrates an anti-inflammatory effect 30x more potent than hydrocortisone, however, at the expense of zero mineralocorticoid effect. Dexamethasone is not a preferred treatment with Addison's disease as the strong effect may lead to Cushing's syndrome, and require a concurrent increased dosage of fludrocortisone.

#17. c) The maturation of the Zona Reticularis
Adrenarche refers to the maturation of the zona reticularis of the adrenal gland, prevalent around ages 6-8 years. It may overlap with puberty; however, this is not dependent upon functional gonads – the process of adrenarche is adrenal dependent and may occur in the presence of hypogonadism. With adrenarche, patients demonstrate pubic hair, sebaceous and apocrine gland synthesis. Weak androgens such as Dehydroepiandrosterone (DHEA) are released from the zona reticularis.

#18. d) Inactivates Cortisol to Cortisone
11-beta hydroxysteroid dehydrogenase type II is prominent near the mineralocorticoid receptors and renal tissue, which inactivates cortisol to cortisone; 11-beta hydroxysteroid dehydrogenase type I is prevalent within the liver, functioning to re-activate cortisone to cortisol. In addition to genetic mutations of the gene coding for the enzyme, liquorice, carbenoxolone and tobacco are known to inhibit the enzyme. Moreover, ectopic ACTH Syndrome (such as Small-Cell Carcinoma of the Lung) 'saturates' the enzyme, leading to excess cortisol binding to the mineralocorticoid receptors.

#19. e) Expected consequence of the medication
This patient has been taking steroids for a significant period of time, however, is asymptomatic (no infection and unlikely a flare-up of his inflammatory bowel disease). A haematological malignancy would be highly unlikely in and laboratory error, whilst possible, is not the most likely answer. Corticosteroids are known to demonstrate anti-

inflammatory effects, with eosinopaenia (unlike a deficient state of cortisol such as Addison's disease with Eosinophilia), and neutrophilia. Corticosteroids increase release of neutrophils from the bone marrow and detach the 'marginated' form of neutrophils from the endothelium, leading to circulating neutrophils in the absence of infection or inflammation. The patient can be reassured!

<u>#20.</u> a) Diabetes mellitus
Type IV Renal Tubular acidosis is the commonest subtype of RTA, with diabetes mellitus being the most common cause, in addition to lead poisoning, chronic interstitial nephritis, NSAIDs and heparin.

<u>#21.</u> e) Administration of phenoxybenzamine followed by bisoprolol
Alpha-antagonists such as phenoxybenzamine must always be administered before a beta blocker (such as bisoprolol); should a beta blocker be administered first, this leads to a catecholaminergic crisis from unopposed agonism to the alpha receptors with dangerous hypertension. For similar reasons, with cocaine overdose, one must never prescribe beta blockers. A biopsy is not appropriate with a phaeochromocytoma as it will produce a catecholaminergic crisis and may lead to an unnecessary delay in surgical resection. Similarly, rare case-reports have linked dexamethasone suppression tests to the precipitation of a catecholaminergic crisis.

<u>#22.</u> d) 5mg
5mg of Prednisone is equivalent to 20mg of Hydrocortisone – this is important when planning for patients to wean off of steroids.

<u>#23.</u> d) Autoimmune Polyglandular Syndrome Type 2
Autoimmune Polyglandular Syndrome Type II, presenting with the triad of conditions noted above is described as Schmidt Syndrome. Schmidt Syndrome is believed to demonstrate polygenic (and autosomal dominant) inheritance with incomplete penetrance. Type 1 presents with Addison's disease, candidiasis and hypoparathyroidism, inherited in an autosomal recessive fashion. POEMS Syndrome is a rare haematological syndrome describing Polyneuropathy, Organomegaly, Endocrinopathy, Monoclonal protein, and skin changes – this patient purely demonstrates endocrinopathies and is too young to harbour a potential monoclonal protein malignancy (such as multiple myeloma). IPEX Syndrome stands for Immune Dysregulation, Polyendocrinopathy and Enteropathy, X-linked; this condition more commonly affects

males, and this patient (apart from being a female) does not demonstrate an immunodeficient state nor enteropathy.

<u>#24.</u> d) Medication (Iatrogenic)
Cushing's Syndrome is most commonly a result of medication (iatrogenic); following this, pituitary tumours (known as Cushing's Disease) are the most common cause of Cushing's Syndrome. The reverse is also true; the most common cause of an Addisonian crisis is iatrogenic (sudden steroid withdrawal).

<u>#25.</u> a) Phaeochromocytoma
This gentleman is presenting with a medullary thyroid carcinoma and a marfanoid habitus; this is suggestive of Multiple Endocrine Neoplasia Type 2B, an autosomal dominant condition resulting from a mutation in the RET gene. These patients are further at an increased risk for a phaeochromocytoma and intestinal ganglioneuromas (with resultant Hirschsprung's Disease).

<u>#26.</u> d) Continue both medications, however, dosage adjustments are required
During gestation, the dosage of corticosteroids is likely to be increased (including during labour); moreover, progesterone is anti-mineralocorticoid in nature, and many patients will need an increased dose of fludrocortisone. Both hydrocortisone and prednisone are recommended during pregnancy as they are metabolised by 11-beta-hydroxysteroid dehydrogenase type II within the placenta. As this patient is comfortably treated with hydrocortisone, it would be wise to continue the medication. Dexamethasone is not appropriate as this is not metabolised by the placenta; foetuses may demonstrate cleft palate and orofacial clefts.

<u>#27.</u> c) Nelson's Syndrome
This patient had both adrenal glands removed for Cushing's Syndrome; she has since developed Nelson's Syndrome as demonstrated by frequent headaches and hyperpigmentation. When the adrenal glands are removed and the source of Cushing's syndrome is unknown, there is a risk that a pre-existing microadenoma (not identified) will hypertrophy, which is the case with this patient. The hypersecretion of ACTH has led to the pigmentation of this patient.

<u>#28.</u> b) Bisoprolol
Beta-blockers demonstrate a direct inhibition upon the release of renin; therefore, a decrease in the release of renin will result in a falsely elevated ratio of aldosterone-to-renin.

<u>#29.</u> d) Subclinical Cushing's Syndrome
Amongst incidentalomas, up to 15% may demonstrate the release of cortisol – this may not be clinically obvious (known as Subclinical Cushing's Syndrome). Treatment is individualised for the patient; despite the absence of overt symptomatology, the excess cortisol nonetheless is minacious. Less commonly, the 'incidentaloma' may demonstrate the release of aldosterone (Conn's Syndrome) or catecholamines (Phaeochromocytoma). Rapid-onset virilisation is concerning for an adrenal carcinoma; however, this is very uncommon. Moreover, SIADH is not a result of an 'incidentaloma' but may occur with a renal-cell-carcinoma.

<u>#30.</u> b) Overnight Dexamethasone Suppression Test (1mg)
The dexamethasone suppression test is the preferred investigation to assess for subclinical Cushing's syndrome with an adrenal 'incidentaloma'. Following an uncertain or equivocal result, the 8mg Dexamethasone Suppression test is performed for confirmation. Urinary Free Cortisol is not performed due to its low accuracy with subclinical Cushing's syndrome – by the time a urinary free cortisol investigation becomes positive the disorder is more advanced. It is important to note that plasma cortisol and ACTH on their own are labile and a single 'random' test of either does not prove or disprove the diagnosis. Although extremely uncommon, one must be cautious if there is a chance the mass is a phaeochromocytoma, as certain medications (including dexamethasone) have been noted to precipitate a catecholaminergic crisis.

<u>#31.</u> c) Classic congenital adrenal hyperplasia
Testicular Adrenal Rest Tumours (TARTs) are believed to occur from abnormal migration of primitive germ cells from the mesodermal ridge; cells targeted for adrenal cortical function end-up travelling with primitive gonadal tissue and arrive in the testis. Excessive ACTH release (as with Classic Congenital Adrenal Hyperplasia) leads to hypertrophy of the tissue, and the appearance of bilateral testicular masses, often confused for Leydig-Cell Tumours. 'TARTs' are uncommon with non-classic congenital adrenal hyperplasia. Apart from classic congenital

adrenal hyperplasia, TARTs have furthermore been noted with Cushing's Disease and Nelson's Syndrome. For reasons that are unknown, females with classic congenital adrenal hyperplasia rarely demonstrate ovarian adrenal rest tumours.

#32. d) Phaeochromocytoma
In normal gestation, supine position leads to aorto-caval compression and resultant hypotension. With a phaeochromocytoma, however, when lying supine, the gravid uterus may compress the phaeochromocytoma, leading to the release of catecholamines and paradoxical supine hypertension. This may be confused with pre-eclampsia or gestational hypertension.

#33. a) Ketoconazole
Ketoconazole, Mitotane, Etomidate and Metyrapone are medications occasionally used in Cushing's Syndrome to halt cortisol synthesis. Mifepristone, a glucocorticoid receptor antagonist, does not inhibit cortisol synthesis, but rather can be used to improve hypertension and diabetes in patients with Cushing's Syndrome (this is not readily available as it is an abortifacient in females).

#34. a), c) and d) (option e)
Tobacco, Liquorice and Carbenoxolone all inhibit 11-beta hydroxysteroid dehydrogenase type II, preventing inactivation of cortisol to cortisone.

#35. a) Postural Test
This test is not performed in clinical practice, however, is still popular amongst medical school exams! An adrenal adenoma is more strongly under the influence of ACTH, whereby bilateral adrenal hyperplasia is not (intact renin-angiotensin-aldosterone system). Plasma Aldosterone Concentration is measured at 8AM (after an overnight supine sleep), followed by levels measured at noon (after four hours of being upright). As ACTH levels are highest upon awakening, by lunchtime they reach a nadir, therefore the plasma aldosterone concentration will be decreased with Conn's Syndrome. With Bilateral Adrenal Hyperplasia, the erect posture of the patient for four hours will lead to a compensatory increase in plasma aldosterone concentration.

<u>#36.</u> b) Glucocorticoids
This patient presents with Glucocorticoid-Remediably Hyperaldosteronism (Familial Hyperaldosteronism), which is characterised by the production of aldosterone partly under the control of ACTH due to gene fusion of 11-beta hydroxylase and aldosterone synthase. Treatment involves corticosteroid administration. Family members must be screened, as there is a severe risk of cerebral aneurysm formation and early-onset strokes.

<u>#37.</u> d) Gynaecomastia
Unilateral Conn's syndrome is best treated with a unilateral adrenalectomy, however, should the patient refuse (or not be a candidate for surgery), mineralocorticoid receptor antagonists are initiated. Spironolactone has the best evidence and is first line; male patients may develop gynaecomastia due to the antiandrogenic effect of the medication, for which they may be switched to eplerenone.

<u>#38.</u> c) Hypokalaemia-induced nephrogenic diabetes insipidus
Although hypokalaemia is not always present in Primary Aldosteronism, when present for a chronic duration, can lead to nephrogenic diabetes insipidus, characterised by increased urination and thirst – the muscle weakness displayed by the gentleman discussed is due to hypokalaemia. Hypertension is unlikely to have caused renal damage with a normal eGFR.

<u>#39.</u> d) Epinephrine
The enzyme Phenylethanolamine N-methyltransferase (PNMT) is present only within the adrenal medulla, responsible for converting norepinephrine to epinephrine, therefore hypersecretion of epinephrine is highly likely to be of adrenal origin (phaeochromocytoma).

<u>#40.</u> e) Dexamethasone
As dexamethasone will not be metabolised by the placenta, this can prevent virilisation of a female foetus, however, this does not change the requirement for lifelong steroid replacement after birth. Virilisation begins by week four, and traditionally chorionic villus biopsy sampling was not available until week 11 when virilisation was complete, therefore dexamethasone would be prescribed until the karyotype of the foetus returned (continued if female, discontinued if male). Currently however, foetal cell-free DNA is becoming more available

across centres, which can detect the karyotype as early as week five. Dexamethasone is administered at 20micrograms/kilogram and is believed to decrease virilisation by nearly 85%. There are risks to the mother (cushingoid appearance, worsened gestational diabetes) and foetus (cleft lip, cleft palate, limited long-term data).

#41. d) Morning
A typical corticosteroid replacement aims for between 15-25mg per day, delivered in two-to-three dosages. As cortisol is highest within the morning, the largest dose is given then. As an example, if a patient is prescribed 20mg of hydrocortisone daily, this would equate to 10mg in the morning, 5mg two hours after lunch and 5mg in the late afternoon. It is important to note that the medication may take up to an hour to have an effect, and therefore when patients wake up, they may feel unwell; for this reason, some physicians advise their patients to set an alarm an hour earlier than when they would usually wake-up and take the dose followed by going back to bed. When they wake up at the designated time, they will already have the mimicked circadian rhythm of high cortisol.

#42. d) Lungs
In particular, small-cell carcinoma of the lungs is notorious for metastasising to the adrenal glands.

#43. a) Perirenal Fat
The renal (perinephric) fascia envelopes both the kidneys and adrenal glands, in addition to anchoring them to the diaphragm. The adrenal glands are separated from the kidneys via the perirenal fat.

#44. b) 5-6 weeks
At around 5-6 weeks gestation, the cortex and medulla of the foetal adrenal gland begin to develop. Mesothelial cells between the mesentery and gonad (urogenital ridge), penetrate mesenchymal tissue to form the inner foetal cortex. At around eight weeks, the outer definitive cortex is formed. The medulla is formed from neural crest cells which begins migration around this time.

#45. b) Foetal Zone; Definitive Zone
The foetal adrenal gland is characterised by the inner 'foetal' and outer 'definitive' zone. During gestation, the majority of the adrenal cortex is

composed of the foetal zone, which predominantly acts to produce sex hormones.

#46. b) Achalasia
'Triple A Syndrome' (not to be confused with AAA/Triple A – Abdominal Aortic Aneurysm), is an autosomal recessive condition also known as Allgrove Syndrome. This condition is characterised by Achalasia, Alacrima and ACTH Resistance/Addison's Disease. There are typically neurological sequelae as well such as microcephaly, intellectual disability, and developmental delay. Hyperkeratosis of the hands and feet is a further defining feature. Alacrima is most commonly the first sign, as this is apparent in early life.

#47. d) X-Linked Adrenoleukodystrophy; Lorenzo's Oil
This vignette is characteristic for X-Linked Adrenoleukodystrophy. In the past week, the patient has begun to demonstrate signs of adrenal insufficiency. Lorenzo's Oil is known to decrease the levels of circulating very-long chain fatty acids.

#48. c) Prader-Willi Syndrome; Central Adrenal Insufficiency
This vignette is characteristic of Prader-Willi Syndrome. Apart from paternal imprinting of the gene, another mode of inheritance is uniparental disomy, whereby both copies of chromosome 15 are inherited from the mother. In addition to obesity, short stature, hyperphagia and hypogonadism, there are also endocrine abnormalities, which are a result of hypothalamo-pituitary insufficiency. One such potential complication is central adrenal insufficiency.

#49. a) and c) (option e)
Both Atrial Natriuretic Peptide and Dopamine are known to inhibit the release of aldosterone.

#50. b) Tyrosine Hydroxylase
The enzyme Tyrosine hydroxylase catalyzes the rate-limiting step in the synthesis of catecholamines: Tyrosine hydroxylase converts tyrosine to DOPA, with oxygen, iron and tetrahydrobiopterin as co-factors.

<u>#51.</u> c) Type 2B
von-Hippel Lindau Syndrome (VHL) may be divided into Type 1 (no phaeochromocytoma) and Type 2 (phaeochromocytoma); Type 2 may be further categorised into the following subtypes:
o 2A: Phaeochromocytoma with CNS Haemangioblastoma (no Renal Cell Carcinoma)
o 2B: Phaeochromocytoma with CNS Haemangioblastoma and Renal Cell Carcinoma
o 2C: Phaeochromocytoma only

<u>#52.</u> a) and d) (option e)
Type IV Renal Tubular Acidosis is characterised by Hyporeninaemic Hypoaldosteronism. Spironolactone blocks the effects of aldosterone; however, the serum levels will increase in an attempt to overcompensate. Gordon's Syndrome is also known as Pseudohypoaldosteronism, whereby there is end-resistance to aldosterone, however levels are elevated. Liddle's Syndrome is an activating mutation in the Sodium Channel ENaC, whereby there is hypertension and resultant negative feedback with decreased renin and aldosterone.

<u>#53.</u> a) Weiss Criteria
The Weiss Criteria is a histological scoring system to determine the likelihood of a benign versus malignant incidentaloma of the adrenal gland. Criteria include: Nuclear Grade; Mitotic Rate; Atypical Mitoses; Cytoplasm Character; Architecture of Tumor Cells; Necrosis; Venous Invasion; Sinusoidal Invasion; Tumour Capsular Invasion.

<u>#54.</u> f) Adrenal Insufficiency
With an unremarkable history, this is suggesting that he has normal adrenal function of both glands. All the other options listed are potential complications of a biopsy. In the presence of a solitary functioning adrenal gland, then adrenal insufficiency is a major potential complication and biopsy is best avoided, however, this is not the case.

<u>#55.</u> a) Cannot distinguish carcinoma from adenoma
A biopsy of an incidentaloma cannot distinguish carcinoma from an adenoma; although it may be able to distinguish an adrenal lesion from a metastasis, this is unlikely to change the management plan as one is likely already aware of the primary cancer's origin.

#56. b) Collision Tumour
A collision tumour is defined at two histologically distinct, adjacent neoplasms within the adrenal gland.

#57. a) Amitriptyline
Tricyclic Antidepressants, such as Amitriptyline, must be withheld prior to a 24-hour urinary collection of catecholamines, as this will result in a falsely elevated urinary catecholamine measurement. All of the other medications listed are known to decrease the levels of urinary catecholamines.

#58. b) X-Linked Adrenoleukodystrophy
This is an x-linked disorder (male patients) in which there may be concurrent neuro-adrenal damage as a result of circulating very-long-chain fatty acids.

#59. a) Autoimmune Polyglandular Syndrome Type 1
Autoantibodies to Interferon-Omega may be demonstrated in Autoimmune Polyglandular Syndrome Type 1.

#60. a) Dehydroepiandrosterone 25-50mg
The adrenal gland is a prominent source of androgens for females, therefore in adrenal insufficiency they may be eligible for a six-month trial of DHEA (Dehydroepiandrosterone) 25-50mg. DHEAs (Dehydroepiandrosterone-Sulphate) is used as a measurement of the efficacy of DHEA (measured prior to the morning dose being administered).

#61. c) 25%
Congenital Adrenal Hyperplasia is inherited in an autosomal recessive pattern. With both parents' carriers, there is a 1/2x1/2 chance that a child will inherit both healthy copies (1/4 or 25% healthy). Moreover, there is a 1/2x1/2 chance that both mutated copies are inherited (1/4 or 25% affected) and there is a 1/2 (50%) chance that the patient will be a carrier.

#62. e) No treatment is recommended
In asymptomatic male patients, no treatment is typically recommended for non-classic Congenital Adrenal Hyperplasia.

#63. a) Combined Oral Contraceptive Pills
Urinary Free Cortisol measures the 'free'/filtrated portion within the serum and hence is not affected by oestrogen-containing compounds (which increase the total, but not free cortisol levels within the serum). All other options listed are known to affect the accuracy of the test.

#64. b) and c) (option e)
Nephrotic Syndrome will lead to a loss of proteins and hence a falsely lowered 'total' cortisol level as the assay measures the total serum cortisol. Low-dose dexamethasone suppression testing is recommended in renal failure and in an adrenal incidentaloma.

#65. d) Cushing's Disease refers to a pituitary mass, whereas Cushing's Syndrome is an umbrella term for any cause of Cushing's
The terms are not interchangeable – Cushing's Disease is a result of a pituitary microadenoma, whereas the umbrella term for any cushingoid appearance is known as Cushing's Syndrome.

#66. c) Bartter's Syndrome
Bartter's Syndrome is an autosomal recessive disorder, characterised by a mutation in the Na-K-2Cl receptor. This syndrome is akin to an intrinsic loop-diuretic. There will be resultant renin and aldosterone secretion in an attempt to elevate the blood pressure.

#67. e) Incidentaloma and concurrent essential hypertension
The laboratory panel demonstrates increased renin and aldosterone, which is therefore against a diagnosis of Conn's Syndrome. Moreover, there is a normal response to dexamethasone, and normal catecholamine metabolites within the urine. This is therefore likely to be a benign incidentaloma, with concurrent hypertension (essential).

#68. b) and d) (option e)
This vignette is descriptive for The Carney Complex, which is an autosomal dominant disorder characterised by multi-organ involvement and tissue overgrowth. It is a result of a mutation in the tumor suppressor gene PKAR1-alpha, which regulates Protein-Kinase A activity). This syndrome is associated with cardiac myxoma, spotted pigmentation of the skin, café au lait spots, and varying endocrinological abnormalities, the commonest being Primary Pigmented Nodular Adrenocortical Disease (PPNAD). PPNAD is characterised by multiple micronodular lesions on the adrenal gland

which are pigmented. PPNAD demonstrates Cushing's syndrome; the pathophysiology is incompletely understood but is believed to be associated with the presence of adrenal-stimulating antibodies.

<u>#69.</u> c) Cardiac Myxoma
Cardiac Myxomas are characteristic of the Carney Complex, present in up to 60% of those affected. They may occur in any chamber of the heart and may occur synchronously. These are often recurrent; it is estimated that up to 10% of cardiac myxomas in the population are due to underlying Carney Complex.

<u>#70.</u> e) and f) (option h)
Macronodular Adrenal Hyperplasia is often confused with PPNAD; however, the former is more common amongst older patients. The histological description of atrophy between nodules is characteristic for PPNAD, as is the CT sign of 'string of beads appearance'. Whilst PPNAD is associated with the Carney Complex, Macronodular Adrenal Hyperplasia is associated with McCune-Albright Syndrome, Multiple Endocrine Neoplasia Type 1 and Familial Adenomatous Polyposis. A paradoxical increase in cortisol during the Liddle Test is characteristic for PPNAD. Finally, Macronodular Adrenal Hyperplasia is often demonstrated to harbour aberrant hormone receptors, such as Gastric Inhibiting Polypeptide, Catecholamines and Luteinising Hormone (to name a few).

<u>#71.</u> c) and e) (option f)
A carotid body tumour (chemodectoma) is a parasympathetic paraganglioma. As with most parasympathetic paragangliomas, they are silent (non-secretory). Interestingly, these are more common to those living (and born) at high altitudes; moreover, these are more prevalent in females. A classic physical finding on examination is 'Fontaine's Sign', which describes lateral mobility (but poor vertical movement).

<u>#72.</u> e) Organ of Zuckerkandl
The Organ of Zuckerkandl is the only other tissue to carry the enzyme PNMT, which allows for the production of adrenaline. The Organ of Zuckerkandl is derived from chromaffin cells located near the origin of the inferior mesenteric artery.

<u>#73.</u> d) The Carney Triad
The Carney Triad is an extremely uncommon disorder, characterised by Gastrointestinal Stromal Tumours, Paraganglioma and Pulmonary Chondroma. It is currently unknown if the disease is inheritable or not as no genes have been identified; this is in contrast to the Carney-Stratakis Dyad/Syndrome (paraganglioma and gastrointestinal stromal tumour), which is inherited in an autosomal dominant fashion. Some authors view the Carney Triad as its own form of multiple endocrine neoplasia. Other neoplasms encountered may include phaeochromocytoma and adrenocortical adenomas. The Carney Triad is more common in females.

<u>#74.</u> a) Carney-Stratakis Dyad
The Carney-Stratakis Dyad/Syndrome is an autosomal dominant condition characterised by paraganglioma and gastrointestinal stromal tumours. This is characterised by germline mutations of Succinate Dehydrogenase B, C and D.

<u>#75.</u> b) Diabetes Insipidus
A deficiency in corticosteroids (adrenal insufficiency) impairs the clearance of free water; administration of corticosteroids may unmask partial diabetes insipidus.

<u>#76.</u> d) Omeprazole
It is imperative this gentleman is prescribed concurrent gastric protection such as omeprazole, as this high dosage of dexamethasone (similar to NSAIDs) will rapidly lead to peptic ulcer formation.

<u>#77.</u> a) and c) (option d)
Growth Hormone is known to inhibit the enzyme 11-Beta-Hydroxysteroid Dehydrogenase Type 1, which functions to convert cortisone to cortisol. Inhibition of this enzyme with growth hormone replacement may lead to hypocortisolism and therefore the dosage may need to be increased. Moreover, concurrent growth hormone and corticosteroid administration worsens serum glucose levels.

<u>#78.</u> d) Transdermal oestrogen has no effect upon total cortisol
Oral oestrogen induces the liver to increase cortisol-binding-globulin (CBG) and hence may lead to an elevated 'total' cortisol measurement. This is not seen with transdermal oestrogen.

#79. d) (1) Is the mass benign or malignant; (2) Is the mass functional or non-functional
The two most important aspects when assessing an adrenal incidentaloma are the risk of malignancy, and secretory status.

#80. d) 70-90%
The vast majority of adrenal incidentalomas are silent, however, of the remaining 'active' lesions, the majority produce cortisol (subclinical cushing's syndrome), followed by aldosterone and catecholamines.

#81. d) Phaeochromocytoma
Growth-Hormone-Releasing Hormone (GHRH) can be released from a phaeochromocytomas (and other neuroendocrine tumours) leading to paraneoplastic acromegaly.

#82. a) or b) (option d)
Primary aldosteronism may improve in a certain percentage of patients during pregnancy as the levels of progesterone increase and function as mineralocorticoid antagonists. Other patients may demonstrate worsening of the disease, as a result of luteinising-hormone choriogonadotrophin receptor expression within the adenomas.

#83. d) Administer three-times usual daily dose for three days; seek medical attention if no improvement by day four
There is no need to go to the hospital for a minor illness unless the patient does not have enough medication. For a minor illness such as an upper respiratory tract infection and minor fever, the three-by-three rule may be applicable, with 3x the daily dosage for three days.

#84. c) and d) (option e)
Hypoglycaemia is much less common in adult patients presenting with an Addisonian crisis or adrenal insufficiency than children. Moreover, secondary adrenal insufficiency is more likely to harbour hypoglyaemia due to the potential for other hormone deficiencies such as growth hormone and thyroid-stimulating hormone (hyperthyroidism worsens glycemia control).

#85. b) 21-hydroxylase
Autoantibodies directed towards 21-hydroxylase are present in the majority of patients with addison's disease. Antibody titres will decline

over time and are highest at diagnosis. Moreover, antibodies are proportional to the degree of adrenal dysfunction.

#86. d) Decrease salt intake
In the presence of co-existing primary hyperaldosteronism and primary hypertension, salt intake should be minimised, and the dose of fludrocortisone may need to be decreased (but not avoided!).

#87. a) and b) (option d)
Various medications may interfere with the uptake of MIBG leading to spurious results; for this reason, a medication history is very important. Other medications include:
> *o Opioids*
> *o Beta-Blockers*
> *o Amiodarone*
> *o Salbutamol*
> *o Calcium Channel Blockers*
> *o ACE-Inhibitors*

#88. e) All of the above
The serum aldosterone-renin ratio becomes unreliable in the presence of hypokalaemia due to its inhibitory effect upon aldosterone release. Hypokalaemia and blood pressure are to be corrected prior to the test; moreover, NSAIDs will lead to a false positive result by reducing renin and increasing aldosterone. Renal failure will inevitably lead to hyperreninaemia and this test will be unreliable. Finally, advances age is associated with a falsely elevated increase in the ratio (renin lowered more than aldosterone), limiting the usefulness of the test and therefore many authors propose a higher cut-off for elderly patients.

#89. d) Central Pontine Myelinolysis; Saline
Rapid over-correction of chronic hyponatraemia may lead to Central Pontine Myelinolysis (Osmotic Demyelination Syndrome) leading to absence of osmolytes and causing both pontine and extra-pontine neurones (such as oligodendrocytes) to shrink, with resultant demyelination. This vignette suggests the patient has a history of poor adherence to medication and likely has chronic hyponatraemia. Rapid correction may lead to dysphagia, paralysis, dysarthria, pseudobulbar palsy and the potential for locked-in syndrome, and death.

<u>#90.</u> d) Selective Adrenal Venous Sampling
A CT or MRI will not identify all lesions within the adrenal gland; lesions below 1cm in diameter can be easily missed. Selective Adrenal Venous Sampling is suggested in this vignette as it can determine the size of the lesion if unilateral. Furthermore, unilateral disease can be managed with surgery, whereby bilateral disease is managed with spironolactone.

<u>#91.</u> c) n-myc
n-myc is a proto-oncogene which is typically amplified in a neuroblastoma and associated with a worse prognosis.

<u>#92.</u> b) Sephardic Jews (Moroccan Ancestry)
Jewish people of Moroccan Ancestry have an increased prevalence of this disorder, which may be due to a founder effect.

<u>#93.</u> c) Phaeochromocytoma
Beckwith-Wiedemann Syndrome may present with hemihypertrophy, macroglossia, hypoglycaemia, omphalocoele (amongst many signs), in addition to an increased risk of malignancies. On such malignancy with an increased prevalence amongst patients with Beckwith-Wiedemann Syndrome is a phaeochromocytoma. Other malignancies include Wilm's Tumour (Nephroblastoma) and Hepatoblastoma.

<u>#94.</u> e) All of the above
Chromogranin A is co-released with gastrin, and therefore in situations such as pernicious anaemia, proton-pump inhibitors and post-ingestion, both levels will inevitably be elevated. Moreover, there is a risk of a false positive form heterophile antibody interference with serum assays.

<u>#95.</u> c) Dexamethasone
*Dexamethasone is used for screening tests as it is **not** detected by assay measurements.*

<u>#96.</u> d) 100-150 micrograms
100-150 micrograms of aldosterone are released from the adrenal cortex each day; this is why patients with primary adrenal insufficiency (not secondary or tertiary adrenal insufficiency) require 100-150micrograms of fludrocortisone replacement.

#97. c) Multiple Endocrine Neoplasia Type 1
Conn's Syndrome has very rarely been associated with Multiple Endocrine Neoplasia Type 1.

#98. c) Decline in the release of dehydroepiandrosterone (DHEA) and dehydroepiandrosterone-sulfate (DHEA-s) with increasing age
Adrenopause (distinct to Andropause) refers to the decrease in release of the androgens from the zona reticularis of the adrenal cortex, as a consequence of normal ageing.

#99. c) Adrenocortical Carcinoma; Li-Fraumeni Syndrome
Li-Fraumeni syndrome is due to an inactivating mutation in the tumour suppressor gene p-53, and is associated with breast cancer, sarcomas, leukaemia and adrenocortical carcinomas.

#100. b) Hypercalcaemia
Addison's Disease is associated with a mild hypercalcaemia; however, the underlying reason is not known. Multiple theories include volume contraction, increased tubular reabsorption, decreased glomerular filtration and increased protein-binding.

<u>Thyroid Gland</u>

#1. A 33-year-old female patient with a background of Hashimoto's Thyroiditis presents to the endocrine clinic for a six-week follow-up after commencing levothyroxine (1.6 micrograms/kg). Her medical history is only significant for fibroids and a history of gestational diabetes with her prior pregnancy. At the current appointment, she reports no improvement of her symptoms, and her blood results demonstrate the following:

Free T4	8.0pmol/L (Ref: 12-22pmol/L)
Thyroid-Stimulating Hormone	6.0mU/L (Ref: 0.27-4.2mU/L)

What is the most likely reason for her lack of improvement both clinically and biochemically?
- a) Medication interaction
- b) Non-compliance
- c) Antithyroxine autoantibodies
- d) Dosage is too low

#2. In the absence of underlying thyroid disease, administration of which of the following vitamins lead to assay interference, with resultant test results resembling hyperthyroidism?
- a) B1
- b) B7
- c) Folate
- d) Vitamin C

#3. A 16-year-old female is followed up by her psychiatrist after experiencing her third manic episode in five years, despite compliance with Sodium Valproate and Olanzapine. The psychiatrist is keen to initiate Lithium for Bipolar Disorder Type I, however, the patient is worried as she has read online that Lithium 'damages your kidneys'. Her psychiatrist emphasises that she will be frequently followed up through appointments and blood tests, monitoring her renal function and which of the following other tests?
- a) Liver Function Tests
- b) Thyroid Function Tests
- c) Lipid Levels
- d) Creatine Kinase
- e) Bone Profile (Calcium, Phosphate and Parathyroid Hormone)

#4. A junior doctor at the local training hospital has been asked to give a lecture to the first-year medical students regarding thyroid hormone synthesis. Whilst reviewing the hormonal synthesis pathway taking place within the thyroid gland, an astute student in the first row asks what the recommended daily intake of iodine is for a non-pregnant adult. Which of the following is the correct response?

    a) 150 milligrams
    b) 200 micrograms
    c) There is no minimum daily intake recommended
    d) 200 milligrams
    e) 150 micrograms

#5. After answering the student's query in question #4, the discussion of thyroid hormone synthesis is continued. The junior doctor discusses the importance of thyroglobulin, which is formed in the rough endoplasmic reticulum and transported into the follicular lumen. Iodine is attached to tyrosine residues on thyroglobulin through the enzyme thyroid peroxidase, creating both monoiodotyrosine and diiodotyrosine (which are further combined to create T3 and T4). The junior doctor asks the lecture hall in which of the following clinical situations would a physician measure serum thyroglobulin level?

    a) Suspicion for Papillary Carcinoma
    b) Recurrence of medullary thyroid carcinoma
    c) Factitious Hyperthyroidism
    d) Recurrence of Papillary Carcinoma
    e) c) and d)

#6. Which of the following best describes the hormone triiodothyronine (T3)?

    a) 80% is produced by the thyroid gland
    b) 100% is produced by the thyroid gland
    c) 80% is produced by the deiodinase enzymatic system in the periphery
    d) T3 is not produced in the thyroid gland
    e) None of the above are correct

#7. A primigravida presents for her neonatal well-being appointment, with an estimated gestational age of 10 weeks. Her only past medical history is significant for common migraines (migraines without aura); however, she does not take any medication for this. Her remaining medical history is unremarkable apart from a family history of her mother and sister both suffering with Graves' Disease. Her only concern at the moment is of variable morning nausea and vomiting and occasional headaches. As per local hospital policy you order a full blood count, renal function and electrolytes, hepatitis titre and thyroid function tests. The laboratory technician notifies you to flag up an abnormal result, demonstrated below:

Total T4	24pmol/L (Ref: 4.5-10.9 micrograms/dL/L)
Thyroid-Stimulating Hormone	0.23mU/L (Ref: 0.27-4.2mU/L)
Free T4	16pmol/L (12-22pmol/L)

Which of the following is the most likely diagnosis?

- a) Hyperemesis Gravidarum
- b) Pre-eclampsia
- c) Subclinical Hyperthyroidism
- d) Graves' Disease
- e) Normal gestational phenomenon

#8. The father of a three-year old child brings his son in for a same-day appointment after noticing a lump in his neck. He is very concerned this could be leukaemia, as his older sister was diagnosed with Acute Lymphoblastic Leukaemia four years ago, however, she is currently in remission. The vital signs of the child are satisfactory, and he appears to play with the toy truck with content. Other than the 'common flu' three weeks ago, his medical history is unremarkable. When examining the child, the mass is noted to be located in the midline of the neck, is non-tender and mobile. You ask the father to make a silly face, and as the boy copies (sticking his tongue out), you note the mass elevates upwards. The father should be informed that:

- a) Urgent chemotherapy is required
- b) The diagnosis is a thyroglossal duct cyst
- c) He is unlikely to harbour functioning thyroid tissue
- d) A sistrunk procedure may be performed for the condition
- e) b) and d)

#9. Graves' disease can be treated medically, surgically or with radiological intervention. Should a patient be treated with either Carbimazole or Propylthiouracil, in addition to the risk for potential hepatotoxicity, which of the following is true regarding thionamide medications?

a) The oral contraceptive pill will become unreliable
b) One cannot become pregnant on these medications due to the severe teratogenicity
c) In the presence of a sore throat or fever, discontinue the medication and seek urgent medical attention
d) Although a rash may occur, there is no risk for drug-induced vasculitis
e) Both Propylthiouracil and Carbimazole are pro-drugs

#10. Which of the following medications contains 37% iodine, and hence may lead to both hypothyroidism and hyperthyroidism?
a) Amiodarone
b) Lithium
c) Eplerenone
d) Tocilizumab
e) Aripiprazole

#11. A newlywed couple present to their general practitioner. They would like to begin a family, however, are concerned about the safety of pregnancy, as the wife suffers with Hashimoto's Thyroiditis. She asks if it is safe to continue her levothyroxine dosage, or if she should discontinue the medication. Which of the following is the best advice to deliver to the couple?
a) Levothyroxine is teratogenic
b) Levothyroxine dosage must be continued, but at a lower dosage
c) Levothyroxine must be switched to Liothyronine
d) Levothyroxine must be continued, but at an increased dose
e) Levothyroxine must be continued, with the addition of Liothyronine

#12. During embryogenesis, the thyroid gland is the first endocrine organ to develop. The thyroid of the foetus is able to commence hormonal synthesis by 12 weeks' gestation. Which of the following demonstrates the origin of development of the thyroid gland?
a) Tuberculum impar
b) Copula

c) Foramen Caecum
d) Foramen Appendicum
e) Trachea

#13. The thyroid gland, in addition to the follicular cells, contains the parafollicular C-cells, derived from the ultimobranchial bodies. From which pharyngeal pouch do the ultimobranchial bodies develop from?
a) First pharyngeal pouch
b) Second pharyngeal pouch
c) Third pharyngeal pouch
d) Fourth pharyngeal pouch
e) Fifth pharyngeal pouch

#14. A 34-year-old male is under close observation from a clinical endocrinologist. He is known to harbour a mutation in the RET gene. His mother developed both hyperparathyroidism and a phaeochromocytoma. Which of the following neoplasms is he further at risk for developing?
a) Insulinoma
b) Glucagonoma
c) Laryngeal Papilloma
d) Medullary Thyroid Carcinoma
e) Parathyroid Carcinoma

#15. A 36-year-old Veterinarian is referred to the endocrinology department. She had demonstrated palpitations, chest pain and anxiety, for which her general practitioner requested free T4 and TSH. Her family history is significant for Graves' disease in her father and brother. She denies any headaches or weight loss and no exophthalmos is noted on examination. She lives alone, with two cats and a dog. The general practitioner is very concerned, and asks for a pituitary MRI after the following results:

Free T4	24pmol/L (Ref: 12-22pmol/L)
Thyroid-Stimulating Hormone	5.1.0mU/L (Ref: 0.27 4.2mU/L)

Which of the following is the likely diagnosis?
a) TSHoma (Pituitary Adenoma)
b) Heterophile Antibody Interference
c) Subclinical Hyperthyroidism
d) Refetoff (Thyroid hormone Resistance) Syndrome
e) Subclinical Hypothyroidism

#16. Calcitonin, a hormone functioning to decrease serum calcium, can be used as a tumour marker for recurrence of which neoplasm?
- a) Medullary Thyroid Carcinoma
- b) Thyroid Paraganglioma
- c) Parathyroid Carcinoma
- d) Anaplastic Carcinoma
- e) Lymphoma

#17. Which of the following is the biggest risk factor for both Graves' Disease and Ophthalmopathy (nearly doubles the risk)?
- a) Alcohol
- b) Type A Personality
- c) Pregnancy
- d) Smoking
- e) Ethnicity

#18. Many infections promote 'molecular mimicry', whereby antibodies formed towards the infection self-attack human tissues. Which of the following infections is believed to promote molecular mimicry (and hence Graves' Disease)?
- a) Yersinia Pestis
- b) Escherichia Coli
- c) Yersinia Entercolitica
- d) Malaria
- e) Syphilis

#19. A 17-year-old female presents with an irregular heartbeat, which is confirmed as atrial fibrillation. She has noted weight loss, diarrhoea, amenorrhoea and a tremor. She is not too concerned with her symptoms, as she believes this is due to the stress over applying to universities. There is no family history of thyroid disease, and there is an absence of exophthalmos and goitre on physical examination. She does complain however, that she feels more 'bloated' than usual, and her abdomen is mildly distended on examination. Select the most likely diagnosis:
- a) Factitious Hyperthyroidism
- b) Amphetamine Abuse
- c) Normal Anxiety
- d) Struma Ovarii
- e) Coeliac's Disease

#20. A multigravida G4P3 gives birth to a male infant at 40 weeks' gestation. His APGAR scores were 9 and 10 at one and ten minutes, respectively. Gestational history was significant only for Hashimoto's Thyroiditis. On the second day post-partum, the parents note a 'bald patch' on the infant's head. The most likely diagnosis and its respective cause are:

    a) Aplasia Cutis; Levothyroxine Therapy
    b) Aplasia Cutis; Carbimazole
    c) Hyperplasia Cutis; Carbimazole
    d) Hypertrophia Cutis; Propylthiouracil
    e) Aplasia Cutis; Bisoprolol

#21. A group of medical students are shadowing the attending physician in the endocrine ward. The medical students would like to know if there are any other physical signs (apart from ophthalmopathy) which may suggest the diagnosis of Graves' Disease. Which of the following is a physical sign specific for Graves' Disease?

    a) Hyperpigmentation of the upper eyelid
    b) Acropachy
    c) Pretibial Myxoedema
    d) Thyroid Bruit
    e) All of the above

#22. Which of the following minerals is believed to decrease autoantibody titres, promote remission of autoimmune thyroid disease and is a treatment option for mild Graves' Ophthalmopathy?

    a) Manganese
    b) Iodine
    c) Selenium
    d) Magnesium
    e) Zinc

#23. A 65-year-old gentleman undergoes a total thyroidectomy for a suspicious left-lobe lesion. A final year-medical student is offered the chance to 'scrub in' for the surgery. After identifying the pretracheal fascia, the attending surgeon decides to quiz the student. Which of the following correctly identifies the blood supply of the thyroid gland?

    a) Superior Thyroid Artery (branch of Internal Carotid Artery) and Inferior Thyroid Artery (branch of External Carotid Artery)

b)   Superior Thyroid Artery (branch of Subclavian Artery) and Inferior Thyroid Artery (branch of Maxillary Artery)
c)   Superior Thyroid Artery (branch of External Carotid Artery) and Inferior Thyroid Artery (branch of Subclavian Artery)
d)   Superior thyroid Artery (branch of Subclavian Artery) and Inferior Thyroid Artery (branch of Internal Carotid Artery)

#24. A 24-year-old female makes an appointment with her local physician. For the past four months, she has noted weight loss of 2 kilograms (unintentional) despite increasing her caloric intake (insatiable appetite). Her periods have become irregular, and she feels anxious most days (palpitations). Concerned for pregnancy, she has taken three tests, all of which have returned negative. She does not take any prescribed or over the counter medications, nor is there a family history of thyroid disorders. She asks the physician if this could be hyperthyroidism, as her symptoms are very similar to the various blog posts online which she has read. From reviewing the blood results below, the physician is puzzled, and asks for assistance from the local Endocrinology Fellow. Assuming there is no assay interference (artefact), which test should be performed next?

Free T4	20pmol/L (Ref: 12-22pmol/L)
Thyroid-Stimulating Hormone	0.2mU/L (Ref: 0.27-4.2mU/L)

a)   Total T4
b)   eGFR
c)   T3
d)   Urinary Iodine Concentration
e)   Serum Albumin

#25. A 45-year-old businessman, originally from Tokyo, is transported to the emergency department by the paramedics after his wife noted an abnormal behaviour. The wife is concerned the patient has had a stroke – he has been complaining of 'fatigue', muscle weakness and cramping all day, and noted difficulty both sitting down and arising from a chair. Both arms were 'floppy', and he could not support himself. This is very unusual for this patient, who is generally very active and wakes up at 5am to prepare for his business meetings. There is no available family history as he was adopted. His past medical history is significant for a similar episode one month prior, where he became extremely light-headed and unsteady on his feet after having a pint of beer at the pub. He had presumed this was due to alcohol and an erratic eating habit that day. In the emergency department, the following blood results return:

Free T4	35pmol/L (Ref: 12-22pmol/L)
Thyroid-Stimulating Hormone	0.2mU/L (Ref: 0.27-4.2mU/L)
Sodium	145mmol/L (135-145 mmol/L)
Potassium	2.9mmol/L (3.5-5.3mmol/L)
Phosphate	0.7mmol/L (0.74-1.4mmol/L)

Which of the following is the most likely diagnosis?
a) Alcoholic Neuropathy
b) Thyrotoxic Storm
c) Myxoedema Coma
d) Hypokalaemic (Thyrotoxic) Periodic Paralysis
e) Hyperkalaemic (Thyrotoxic) Periodic Paralysis

#26. A patient with long-standing Hashimoto's Thyroiditis would like to find out more about the long-term effects of the disease. Hashimoto's Thyroiditis is a risk factor for development of which of the following?
a) Lymphoma
b) Medullary Carcinoma
c) Papillary Carcinoma
d) a) and c)
e) Anaplastic Carcinoma

#27. A patient reluctantly agrees to commence Carbimazole therapy after a diagnosis of Graves' disease is confirmed. She would like to know for how long she is likely to be treated for with the medication. The correct response is:
a) Lifelong
b) Five years
c) 12-18 months
d) Six Weeks
e) Patient's Choice

#28. The patient is question #27 would like to know if there are any 'scoring systems' that can be used to predict a relapse of her hyperthyroidism. The current scoring system used in clinical practice is:
a) The MATILDA Scoring System

b) The GREAT Score
c) The GRAVE Score
d) The PASS Score
e) Relapse Risk Index

#29. As with most autoimmune conditions, molecular mimicry is believed to be a significant driving factor. Which of the following infections is believed to increase the risk for Hashimoto's thyroiditis?
a) Hepatitis B
b) Hepatitis C
c) Streptococcus Pyogenes
d) Mycobacterium Paratuberculosis
e) Corynebacterium Diphtheria

#30. In a symptomatic patient with a diagnosis of severe hyperthyroidism, the most important class of medication to initiate is:
a) Calcium Channel Blockers
b) Beta-Blockers
c) Thionamides
d) Corticosteroids
e) Levothyroxine

#31. The Wolff-Chaikoff effect is best depicted by which of the following options?
a) Administration of Iodine promotes thyroid hormone release
b) Administration of Iodine promotes thyroid hypertrophy
c) Administration of thyroid hormones promotes iodine synthesis
d) Administration of Iodine inhibits thyroid hormone release
e) Administration of thyroid hormones inhibits the incorporation of Iodine

#32. Karl Adolf von Basedow described the 'Meresburg Triad' in 1840; the components of this triad include Exophthalmos, Goitre and which of the following?
a) Tremor
b) Weight loss
c) Tachycardia

d) Acropachy
e) Pretibial Myxoedema

#33. Although the development of Graves' disease follows a polygenic inheritance, certain 'predisposing factors' have been noted to contribute to the development of the condition. Which of the following is known to increase the risk of acquiring Graves' Disease?
a) HLA-B27
b) HLA-Aw1
c) HLA-DR3
d) CTLA-4
e) c) and d)

#34. With Graves' Ophthalmopathy, which of the following muscles are most severely affected?
a) Lateral Rectus
b) Medial Rectus
c) Inferior Rectus
d) a) and c)
e) b) and c)

#35. Which of the following HLA-Haplotypes is believed to be 'protective' against developing Graves' Disease?
a) HLA-DRB107
b) HLA-DRB108
c) HLA-DRB30101
d) HLA-B3W5
e) All of the above are protective alleles

#36. In patients with Graves' Ophthalmopathy, it is important to classify the findings in order to compare with succeeding follow-up appointments. Which of the following 'scoring systems' may be used to classify and allow follow-up of Graves' Ophthalmopathy?
a) EXOPSPECS
b) Graves Orbitopathy Scoring System
c) NOSPECS
d) Thyroid Eye Questionnaire
e) Rundle's Score

#37. Deficiency of which vitamins is believed to be involved in the pathogenesis of Graves' Disease?

a) Vitamin B1
b) Vitamin D
c) Vitamin B12
d) Vitamin C
e) Vitamin E

#38. Multiple criteria must be fulfilled prior to consideration for a radioiodine ablative procedure as a cure for hyperthyroidism. Which of the following is not an absolute contraindication?
a) Severe Graves' Ophthalmopathy
b) Pre-treatment with thionamides
c) Pregnancy
d) Thyroid Cancer
e) Living at home with children

#39. Which of the following may decrease the success of a radioiodine ablative procedure (likely requiring a second attempt)?
a) Pre-treatment with Lithium
b) Pre-treatment with Carbimazole
c) Pre-treatment with Lugol's Iodine
d) Pre-treatment with Propylthiouracil
e) Pre-treatment with glucocorticoids

#40. For patients requiring a total thyroidectomy, which of the following is a potential complication of the procedure?
a) Recurrent and Superior Laryngeal Nerve transection
b) Hypoparathyroidism
c) Neck Haematoma
d) Thyroid storm
e) All of the above

#41. A 33-year-old female attends her endocrinology appointment with her husband. She was recently diagnosed with Graves' Disease six months ago and is currently prescribed carbimazole. Her and her husband would like to begin a family. She is struggling to take her medications and enquires about alternative treatments. The physician recommends raidioiodine ablation or thyroidectomy. In a female desiring pregnancy, how many months prior should either of these procedures occur?
a) One month

b)   Six Weeks
c)   Six Months
d)   Four Months

#42. Transient neonatal (foetal) thyrotoxicosis occurs when which of the following immunoglobulin (Ig) subtypes cross the placenta?

a)   IgG
b)   IgD
c)   IgB
d)   IgA
e)   IgM

#43. A newborn male is noted to become cyanosed and demonstrates difficulty breathing. Once he begins crying however, the discomfort abates, however the cyanosis returns whilst resting. The paediatric resident is unable to insert a nasogastric tube through either nostril. The paediatric team request radiological imaging, which confirms the diagnosis. Which of the following was the foetus likely exposed to in-utero?

a)   Propranolol
b)   Carbimazole
c)   Atenolol
d)   Levothyroxine
e)   Thyroid Receptor Stimulating Autoantibodies

#44. In a patient from an iodine-deficient region, large administration of iodine (or iodine-containing medications such as amiodarone) may precipitate hyperthyroidism. This is known as:

a)   Wolf-Chaikoff Effect
b)   Jod-Basedow Phenomenon
c)   DeQuervain's Thyroiditis
d)   Graves' Phenomena
e)   None of the above

#45. Within the medical literature, a rare syndrome is occasionally depicted, known as Hirata's Syndrome. This condition is more prevalent in Japanese individuals, with the association of graves' disease, carbimazole and which of the following:

a)   Anti-insulin receptor antibodies
     (hyperglycaemia)
b)   Anti-gliadin antibodies

c) Anti-insulin antibodies (hypoglycaemia)
d) Anti-carbimazole antibodies
e) Anti-T4 antibodies

#46. A 37-year-old male recently married to his college- sweetheart attends the family planning clinic. The couple have been unable to conceive for three years. The female works up comes back unremarkable. A semen analysis and full physical examination are performed for this gentleman, and the results will be delivered to him within the three days. The gentleman's past medical history is significant for recurrent respiratory tract infections, however, and the physician considers cystic fibrosis. A chest x-ray is requested; however, the report suggests right-left reversal (Situs Inversus Totalis). Assuming the birth mother suffered with Graves' disease, which of the following was the gentleman exposed to in-utero?
a) Carbimazole
b) Propranolol
c) IgG autoantibodies
d) Glucocorticoids
e) Propylthiouracil

#47. A 26-year-old male with a known goitre demonstrates engorgement of the facial and neck vessels, in addition to stridor upon demonstration of Pemberton's sign. Moreover, there is dullness to percussion along the anterior sternum. Which of the following is the most likely diagnosis?
a) Superior Vena Cava Syndrome
b) Retrosternal Goitre
c) Ectopic Thyroid Gland
d) Paraneoplastic Syndrome
e) a) and b)

#48. A 24-year-old nursing student is transferred to the emergency department with the paramedics after her partner found her unconscious. For the past three days she has had to miss class due to a severe fever, sweating and diarrhoea. Over the past two months she was noted to demonstrate weight loss and preference for cold, however she presumed this was due to her menstrual cycle. The partner further notes she demonstrated a swelling in her neck at this time but had been too busy to see her general practitioner. On examination the following are noted:

Temperature: 40°C, moist hands
Glasgow Coma Scale: 8/15
Pulse: Irregularly Irregular, 152/minute
Blood Pressure: 162/101mmHg

Which of the following is the most likely diagnosis?

a) Hashitoxicosis
b) Thyroid Storm
c) Sepsis
d) Gastroenteritis
e) None of the above

#49. Which of the following scoring systems can be used to diagnose (and quantify the severity of) a thyroid storm?

a) Wayne's Scoring System
b) Clinical Activity Score
c) Burch and Wartofsky
d) Billewicz Diagnostic Index
e) Zulewski's Clinical Score

#50. Thyroid hormones exist as both protein-bound (majority) and 'free' (active) isoforms. The predominant protein to which thyroid hormones are bound is known as Thyroxine-Binding Globulin (TBG). All of the following are known to increase the TBG except for:

a) Pregnancy
b) Tamoxifen
c) Hepatitis A
d) Androgens
e) Acute Intermittent Porphyria

#51. Fritz de Quervain is credited for the discovery of post-viral thyroiditis in 1904, nowadays referred to as DeQuervain's Thyroiditis. The disorder typically demonstrates three states following an upper respiratory tract infection: Thyrotoxic, Hypothyroid and Euthyroid Phase. Which of the following blood markers is suggestive of DeQuervain's Thyroiditis over Graves' Disease?

a) C-Reactive Protein
b) Erythrocyte Sedimentation Rate (Westergren)
c) Thyroglobulin
d) TSH
e) a) and c)

#52. A 15-year-old female attends family physician with her father. The father explains that his daughter has been complaining of severe palpitations for one month occurring at rest, leading to a sense of anxiety. Throughout the consultation the father does most of the talking, as he explains his daughter suffers from sensorineural hearing loss and has developed recurrent ear infections. The patient is not taking any medications (prescribed or over the counter). The physician notes a very short stature of the patient. Moreover, she seems to be excessively 'fidgety' and unwilling to sit in one position for more than a few seconds. She has been reprimanded at school for failing to pay attention and has been assessed for Attention-Deficit-Hyperactivity disorder. Physical examination demonstrates a prominent lump in the neck, which is non-tender and bilaterally symmetrical, but no other findings of note (no exophthalmos, pretibial myxedema or acropachy). Moreover, a bruit is not present on auscultation of the thyroid gland. A hormonal panel is requested, which demonstrates the following:

Free T4	26pmol/L (Ref: 12-22pmol/L)
Thyroid-Stimulating Hormone	2mU/L (Ref: 0.27-4.2mU/L)
Free T3	7.3pmol/L (Ref: 3.1-6.9pmol/L)

The General Practitioner refers the patient to a consultant endocrinologist, who performs the 'TRH stimulation test', and the TSH begins to increase. Which of the following is the most likely diagnosis?

    a)   Pituitary Adenoma 'TSHoma'
    b)   Illicit substance abuse
    c)   Familial Dysalbuminaemic Hyerthyroxinaemia
    d)   Thyroid Hormone Resistance syndrome
    e)   None of the above

#53. With reference to question #52, if the TRH Stimulation Test failed to increase TSH levels, this may suggest a 'TSHoma'. Which of the following should always be ruled out as a cause of elevated TSH prior to requesting a brain MRI?

    a)   Renal Failure
    b)   Heterophile Antibody Interference
    c)   Serum Albumin
    d)   a) and c)
    e)   a), b) and c)

#54. During a lecture in the endocrinology rotation for final year medical students, the lecturer decides to give a pathological description of a disease and asks the students to name the disorder:

'An autosomal dominant genetic mutation, prevalent amongst Hispanics, whereby albumin abnormally demonstrates a higher capacity for T4 (but not T3). Despite elevated total T4, these patients demonstrate normal free T4, TSH and are clinically euthyroid'. Which of the following is the lecturer describing?

a) Familial Hypoalbuminaemic Thyrotoxicosis
b) Familial Dysalbuminaemic Hypothyroxinaemia
c) Familial Normoalbuminaemic Hyperthyroxinaemia
d) Familial Dysalbuminaemic Hyperthyroxinemia
e) Familial Hyperalbuminaemic Hypothyroxinaemia

#55. Refetoff Syndrome is a clinical disorder whereby there is either pituitary and/or peripheral resistance to thyroid hormones. Pituitary resistance is more likely to demonstrate mild thyrotoxicosis, whereas peripheral resistance may demonstrate hypothyroid symptomatology. The syndrome is characterised by increased free T4 and normal TSH. At times, this may be difficult to differentiate from a TSHoma. Which of the following may be elevated in the serum of patents with a TSHoma?

a) Beta-subunit
b) Gamma-subunit
c) Alpha-subunit
d) Thyroglobulin
e) a) and c)

#56. A 32-year-old female is referred to the neurology department after experiencing an episode of paraesthesia in her left arm. She is otherwise fit and well and does not take any medication. She describes a sensation of 'tingling' that lasted for around two days, before disappearing. She notes this is the second time this has happened, explaining at her 28th birthday she noted the same sensation in her right leg which lasted for two days, but was told this was 'all in her head'. An MRI had been performed, demonstrating diffuse white-plaque formation. Over the next year her condition deteriorates, and she is commenced on a novel monoclonal antibody, targeting CD52, known as Alemtuzumab. One year later, at follow-up, the patient describes feeling hot 'all the time' and is constantly anxious. She is concerned she is going through the menopause, as her mother displayed symptoms of heat intolerance and anxiety when she

went through the menopause at age 48. The physician believes this is an endocrine disorder. Which of the following is the likely diagnosis?
- a) Drug-induced thyroiditis
- b) Drug-induced Graves' Disease
- c) Hyperemesis Gravidarum
- d) Drug-induced hypophysitis

#57. Which of the following antibiotics is known to cause hyperpigmentation of the thyroid gland?
- a) Gentamicin
- b) Penicillin V
- c) Minocycline
- d) Doxycycline
- e) Tazocin

#58. During an audit for first year interns, they decide to review the number of TSH tests ordered. They then decide to compare how many patients with an elevated TSH did not end up having a thyroid disorder. All of the following are known to increase TSH (with normal free T4), except for:
- a) Nephrotic Syndrome
- b) Subclinical Hypothyroidism
- c) Adrenal Insufficiency
- d) Metformin Administration
- e) Age-Related Increase
- f) Obesity

#59. Following Graves' Disease, which of the following is the second most common cause of Hyperthyroidism (particularly prevalent amongst the elderly)?
- a) Multinodular Goitre
- b) TSHoma
- c) Factitious Hyperthyroidism
- d) Medication-induced
- e) DeQuervain's Thyroiditis

#60. In patients hospitalised for severe illness, it is often inappropriate to request a thyroid hormone panel, as it will inevitably return 'abnormal'. In times of severe distress, TSH is known to decrease, with normal T4 and T3 levels. Uniquely, these patients demonstrate increased reverse T3, due to induction of the D3 monodeiodinase enzyme. All of the following options are known to decrease the levels of TSH, except for:

- a) Dopamine, Metformin, Prednisone and Checkpoint Inhibitors
- b) Subclinical Hyperthyroidism
- c) Ethnicity
- d) Central Hypothyroidism
- e) Macro-TSH

#61. In patients treated with anti-epileptic medication, which of the following may be noted if a thyroid hormone panel is requested?

- a) Increased Free T4
- b) Decreased Free T4
- c) Low serum TBG
- d) Increased serum TBG
- e) Suppressed TSH

#62. Heparin may lead to which artefact on a thyroid hormone panel?

- a) Decreased binding of T3 to TBG
- b) Decreased binding of T4 to albumin
- c) Decreased binding of T3 to albumin
- d) Decreased binding of T4 to TBG
- e) b) and d)

#63. In patients with severe neck discomfort, who are suffering from DeQuervain's Thyroidits, which of the following correctly identifies the sequences of medications to be initiated?

- a) Aspirin; Carbmiazole
- b) Carbimazole; Prednisone
- c) Prednisone; Aspirin
- d) Aspirin; Prednisone
- e) Carbimazole; Aspirin

#64. Which of the following haplotypes is linked with the development of DeQuervain's Thyroiditis?

- a) HLA-B36
- b) HLA-B35
- c) HLA-B34
- d) HLA-D35
- e) HLA-D36

#65. A 32-year-old primigravida gives birth to a healthy female infant at 39 weeks' gestation. There are no concerns at the follow-up appointments. Five months later the mother presents to her general practitioner with complains of lethargy, weight loss and secondary amenorrhoea. Her blood results demonstrate the following:

Free T4	11pmol/L (Ref: 12-22pmol/L)
Thyroid-Stimulating Hormone	0.1mU/L (Ref: 0.27-4.2mU/L)
IGF-1	20nmol/L (Ref: 13-33nmol/L)

An MRI of the pituitary demonstrates stalk enhancement. Which of the following is the most likely diagnosis?

- a) Sheehan's Syndrome
- b) van-Wyck-Grumbach Syndrome
- c) Lymphocytic Hypophysitis
- d) Empty Sella Syndrome

#66. A 22-year-old engineering student with a three-year history of autoimmune hypothyroidism presents to her family physician for follow-up. She has been up titrated to a current dose of 400 micrograms/day of levothyroxine, however, is continuing to demonstrate lethargy and malaise. There are no obvious anomalies on physical examination. Family history is contributory for a younger sister suffering with Type 1 Diabetes Mellitus. A hormonal panel is demonstrated below:

Free T4	10pmol/L (Ref: 12-22pmol/L)
Thyroid-Stimulating Hormone	12mU/L (Ref: 0.27-4.2mU/L)

What is the most likely cause for persistently elevated TSH despite being prescribed thyroxine therapy?

- a) Dosage is too low
- b) Malabsorption
- c) Non-compliance (Pseudomalabsorption)
- d) Medication interaction

#67. The patient in question #66 demonstrates adherence, and her partner vouches for her that she takes her medication in the early morning an hour before having breakfast. The patient undergoes a T4-absorption test under clinical supervision. The patient fasts overnight and returns to the clinic the following morning and is observed taking 1,000 micrograms of levothyroxine. The TSH level does not alter, and the free T4 fails to increase at 0, 30, 45 and 120 minutes. Which of the following will confirm the most likely diagnosis?

- a) Anti-tissue transglutaminase antibody

b)   Saccharomyces Cerevisiae antibody
c)   pANCA
d)   ESR
e)   CRP

#68. For patients demonstrating poor adherence with daily levothyroxine, which of the following is approved by the American Thyroid Association as a method to increase the likelihood of adherence?

a)   Once-monthly injection
b)   Once-weekly injection
c)   Once-weekly oral ingestion
d)   Once-monthly oral ingestion
e)   a) and c)

#69. The administration of levothyroxine must be a slow and gradual increment. For elderly patients, there is concern of higher dosages precipitating/worsening which of the following?

a)   Erectile Dysfunction
b)   Breast Tenderness
c)   Atrial fibrillation
d)   Angina Pectoris
e)   c) and d)

#70. It is important to note that some patients may demonstrate persistent symptoms of hypothyroidism despite biochemical euthyroidism – this may occur in up to 10% of patients. The predominant symptoms are tiredness, decreased quality of life, altered mood and 'brain fog'. These patients are believed to harbour either a qualitative or quantitative defect in the enzyme Type 2 Deiodinase, limiting the conversion of T4 to T3. Many of these patients are note an improved quality of life and psychometric performances when prescribed as a combination medication. Due to the limited evidence however, genetic testing for a mutation within the DIO2 gene is not currently recommended. Which of the following is an absolute contradiction to the initiation of liothyronine (LT3) combination therapy?

a)   Elderly patients
b)   Pregnancy
c)   Liver failure
d)   Renal Failure

e) Mild Arrhythmia

#71. A three-year-old child, recently immigrated to Canada with his mother from South America, is noted to be lethargic, constantly tired, and gaining weight. A hormonal panel demonstrates lowered T4 and T3 levels, and elevated TSH. A diagnosis of hypothyroidism is confirmed. Of note however, on performing a physical examination, there is no goitre. Family history is negative for any thyroid disorders. The child is commenced on levothyroxine and is followed up, however at three months there is still no improvement. During a second physical examination, the physician notes a large haemangioma over the left shoulder blade. Which of the following is the most likely diagnosis?

a) Consumptive Hypothyroidism
b) Child Abuse
c) Pseudohypothyroidism
d) Malnutrition
e) b) and d)

#72. Renal failure may induce hypothyroidism by which of the following mechanisms?

a) Albuminuria
b) Loss of free T4
c) Iodine accumulation
d) Iodine depletion
e) None of the above

#73. Iodine deficiency may predispose to which of the following conditions?

a) Thyroid Cancer
b) Goitre
c) Toxic Multinodular Goitre
d) Cretinism
e) All of the above

#74. Approximately what percentage of thyroid 'incidentalomas' are benign?

a) 10-15%
b) 20-30%
c) 50-60%%
d) 90%-95%

> e)   Virtually 100%

#75. The first step in the investigation of a thyroid nodule is which of the following?

> a)   Ultrasound
> b)   Technetium Scan
> c)   Fine Needle Aspiration Biopsy
> d)   Lymph Node Biopsy
> e)   Serum TSH and T4

#76. Thyroid nodules are more prevalent amongst which of the following cohorts?

> a)   Males
> b)   Females
> c)   Iodine-sufficient populations
> d)   Under 40 years of age
> e)   None of the above

#77. A 'red-flag' for which a carcinoma must be suspected as opposed to a benign thyroid nodule includes all of the following except:

> a)   Dysphagia and Stridor
> b)   Rapid Enlargement
> c)   Prior irradiation
> d)   Lymphadenopathy
> e)   Size above two centimetres

#78. Sonography provides vital detail to the echotexture of a thyroid lesion, forming a predominant component of the investigatory pathway. Which of the following findings on a sonogram would be suspicious for a malignant lesion?

> a)   Microcalcifications
> b)   Peripheral Vascularity
> c)   Hypoechoic lesions
> d)   Well-marginated
> e)   a) and c)

#79. Hypothyroidism from Iodine deficiency can be worsened by a concurrent deficit of which of the following vitamins?

> a)   Vitamin C
> b)   Vitamin E
> c)   Vitamin A

d)   Folate
e)   Cyanocobalamin

#80. Which of the following demonstrates a considerable risk reduction in developing Graves' Disease?
a)   Smoking
b)   Severe Emotional Distress
c)   Female Gender
d)   Alcoholism
e)   All of the above

#81. Which of the following disorders is characterised by endometrial cancer, multiple thyroid nodules, nodules on the tongue and invasive ductal breast carcinoma?
a)   von-Hippel Lindau Syndrome
b)   Cowden Syndrome
c)   Cronkhite-Canada Syndrome
d)   Von-Recklinghausen's Disease
e)   Bourneville's Syndrome

#82. All of the following are associated with an increased risk of relapse of Graves' Disease except:
a)   Allergic Rhinitis
b)   Spring and Summer Months
c)   Male gender
d)   Thionamide treatment for five years
e)   Post-partum

#83. A 26-year-old female is referred to the endocrine department with symptomatology suggestive of Graves' Disease. She is noted to demonstrate a palpable, non-tender goitre, resting tachycardia (110 beats per minute), a resting tremor and exophthalmos. She is concerned of the long-term implications of the disorder if she does not get proper treatment? Which of the following options listed below is the commonest (and earliest) sign for Graves' Ophthalmopathy?
a)   Ptosis
b)   Proptosis
c)   Keratitis
d)   Lid-lag
e)   Upper-lid retraction

#84. A 16-year-old female patient presents to her physician with primary amenorrhoea. She is noted to demonstrate a short stature (under 5th centile), a wide-carrying angle and widely spaced nipples. A buccal smear reveals the absence of Barr Bodies. Which of the following conditions is she predisposed to later in life?

- a) Graves' Disease
- b) Autoimmune Hypothyroidism
- c) Lymphocytic Hypophysitis
- d) Thyroid Nodules
- e) Papillary Carcinoma

#85. On physical examination, which of the following signs listed below is suggestive of hypothyroidism?

- a) Thyroid Acropachy
- b) Pretibial Myxoedema
- c) Delayed relaxation of deep tendon reflexes
- d) Central adiposity
- e) None of the above

#86. During a lecture in embryology, the lecturer calls on you to state when in gestation is a foetal thyroid gland is able to produce thyroxine?

- a) 6 weeks
- b) 12 weeks
- c) 16 weeks
- d) 24 weeks
- e) 35 weeks

#87. Which thyroid carcinoma demonstrates 'Orphan Annie Nuclei' on histology?

- a) Follicular Carcinoma
- b) Papillary Carcinoma
- c) Lymphoma
- d) Medullary Carcinoma
- e) Anaplastic Carcinoma

#88. Which of the following thyroid carcinomas spread by the haematogenous route?

- a) Follicular Carcinoma
- b) Papillary Carcinoma
- c) Lymphoma

d) Medullary Carcinoma
e) Anaplastic Carcinoma

#89. In recent years, the medication Ozempic (Semaglutide) has gained attention (and has an FDA Black Box Warning) for the potential to increase the risk of which of the following thyroid neoplasms?
a) Thyroid Paraganglioma
b) Medullary Thyroid Carcinoma
c) Papillary Carcinoma
d) Follicular Adenoma
e) Follicular Carcinoma

#90. The thyroid carcinoma with the worst prognosis is:
a) Follicular Carcinoma
b) Papillary Carcinoma
c) Lymphoma
d) Medullary Carcinoma
e) Anaplastic Carcinoma

#91. Although selenium supplementation is recommended for mild Graves' Ophthalmopathy, which of the following is a potential long-term complication?
a) Type 1 Diabetes Mellitus
b) Acromegaly
c) Type 2 Diabetes Mellitus
d) Cushingoid Appearance
e) Renal Failure

#92. Novel research into Thyroid Associated Ophthalmopathy (TAO) (Graves' Ophthalmopathy) has demonstrated autoantibodies within the fibroblasts and adipocytes of the orbit bind (in addition to TSH Receptors) to Insulin-Like-Growth-Factor 1 (IGF-1) Receptors. IGF-1 receptors are three-to-four times more prevalent in patients with Thyroid Eye Disease compared to normal subjects. The resultant effects include fibroblast stimulation, with deposition of glycosaminoglycans and adipogenesis. Which of the following monoclonal antibodies is a novel treatment which blocks IGF-1 receptors?
a) Tocilizumab
b) Rituximab
c) Telotozumab

d) Teprotumumab
e) Anakinra

<u>#93.</u> What are the two phases of thyroid eye disease?
a) Proliferative and Fibrotic
b) Inflammatory and Fibrotic
c) Hypertrophic and Fibrotic
d) Autoimmune and Fibrotic
e) None of the above

<u>#94.</u> Rundle's Curve is used to graph the natural course of which of the following?
a) Goitre Development
b) Thyroid Eye Disease
c) Autoantibody titres
d) Response to radioiodine treatment
e) None of the above

<u>#95.</u> Up to 50% of patients with Graves' Disease may demonstrate thyroid eye disease manifestations, however, the great majority are not sinister (5% are sight-threatening), with a common endpoint of 'burn out'. Although it is more common in females, severe disease is more likely in male patients. 'Darlymple's Sign is best described as which of the following:
a) Lower lid oedema
b) Unilateral disease
c) Widened palpebral fissure
d) Eyelid tremor
e) Hyperpigmentation of the superior or inferior eyelid

<u>#96.</u> Which of the following ethnicities may demonstrate lower-lid (rather than upper-lid) retraction with Thyroid Eye Disease?
a) Ashkenazic Jews
b) Asians
c) Northern Europeans
d) Afro-Caribbean
e) South Americans

<u>#97.</u> Thyroid Eye Disease (also known as Exophthalmic Goitre or Graves' Orbitopathy), was previously understood to occur as a sole

consequence of Graves' Disease. Recent research, however, has demonstrated this is not wholesome, with Thyroid Eye Disease present with which of the following conditions (apart from Graves' Disease)?

    a) Hashimoto's Thyroiditis
    b) TSHoma
    c) Thyroid Cancer
    d) a) and b)
    e) a) and c)

#98. Sight-threatening Graves' Ophthalmopathy is a medical emergency requiring hospitalisation and the potential for orbital decompressive surgery. Which of the following medications must these patients be administered as an interim?

    a) Intravenous Corticosteroids
    b) Teprotumumab
    c) Mycophenolate Mofetil
    d) Rituximab
    e) Oral Corticosteroids

#99. Four months post-partum, a primigravid 24-year-old presents to her family physician with a six-week history of excess sweating, palpitations and sense of 'overwhelming anxiety'. She is coping at home fine with the baby, and her husband has taken time off of work to spend time with the family. In the past week however, she has begun to feel 'tired all-the-time' and lethargic, with very decreased energy. The family physician is concerned this is a presentation of Post-Partum Thyroiditis, and requests a titre of antithyroid peroxidase, which returns elevated. Which of the following is the most likely clinical outcome?

    a) Permanent Hypothyroidism
    b) Persistent Hyperthyroidism
    c) Euthyroid
    d) Cyclical thyroid disease

#100. The prevalence of a woody, hard and painful thyroid gland, and concurrent retroperitoneal fibrosis should alert a clinician towards which of the following diagnoses?

    a) Riedel's Thyroiditis
    b) Metastatic Renal Cell Carcinoma
    c) Lymphoma

d) IgG4 Disease
e) a) and d)

#101. The natural history of graves' disease in pregnancy is which of the following?

a) Relaxation of symptoms in the first half, followed by aggravation in the second half of pregnancy
b) Aggravation of symptoms in the first half, followed by relaxation in the second half of pregnancy
c) Aggravation of symptoms in the first half, followed by relaxation in the second half of pregnancy; these patients are at an increased risk of relapse post-partum
d) Relaxation of symptoms in the first half, followed by aggravation in the second half of pregnancy; these patients are at a decreased risk of relapse post-partum
e) Relaxation throughout pregnancy, with increased risk of relapse post-partum

#102. The commonest location for ectopic thyroid tissue is which of the following?

a) Lingual Tissue
b) Tonsillar Tissue
c) Pericardium
d) Ovary
e) None of the above

#103. A 26-year-old nurse is followed up by the endocrine department for thyrotoxic symptomatology of six months duration. She has noted occasional palpitations, intolerance to heat and weight loss. There is no family history of thyroid disorders, and her auto-antibody titre of TSH-Receptor Stimulating Antibodies has returned negative on three separate occasions. On physical examination, no goitre is present, and the physician notes an atrophic gland. A thyroid scintigraphy is requested, demonstrating decreased uptake. In the presence of diminished thyroglobulin, the most likely diagnosis is:

a) Thyroiditis
b) Factitious Hyperthyroidism

c) Clinical Anxiety
d) Phaeochromocytoma
e) Struma Ovarii

#104. Hyperemesis-Gravidarum is characterised by excessive (sensitivity or serum levels of) beta-human chorionic gonadotrophin. Patients may present with recurrent, severe nausea, vomiting, ketosis and weight loss. Occasionally, human chorionic gonadotrophin may bind to the TSH receptor, with concurrent negative feedback and decreased TSH. Which of the following options best finishes the following sentence: "______subunit of glycoproteins demonstrates a common origin, whilst ______ subunit of glycoproteins demonstrate specificity:

a) Alpha-subunit; Beta-subunit
b) Beta-subunit; Alpha-subunit
c) Beta-subunit; Gamma-subunit
d) Alpha-subunit; Gamma-subunit
e) Gamma-subunit; Beta-subunit

#105. A 9-year-old boy is brough to the family physician by his mother, who is concerned over the development of multiple brown-patches over his skin. His developmental history is complicated by scoliosis and recurrent skeletal fractures (due to bone replacement by fibrous tissue). In recent weeks, his mother has noted her son to present with severe anxiety, palpitations, intolerance to heat and agitation. She thinks his neck feels enlarged. Which of the following is the likely diagnosis?

a) Carney Complex
b) McCune-Albright Syndrome
c) Pseudohypoparathyroidism
d) Congenital Adrenal Hyperplasia
e) Neurofibromatosis

#106. A 32-year-old PhD Candidate presents to her general practitioner with a four-month history of tiredness and weight gain. She had initially presumed this was due to the 'lack of sleep' over preparing for her dissertation, however, symptoms have worsened despite a proper night's sleep, exercising and healthy dieting. She has never been sexually active, and notes her periods are regular, and there has been no deviation in her regular menstrual pattern over the past four months. She reluctantly admits that two weeks ago she noted a 'whitish discharge' from both nipples, which prompted her to make this appointment. She does not take any prescribed or over-the-counter medications, and there is no family history of endocrinological disorders. Her General Practitioner requests the following:

Free T4	10pmol/L (Ref: 12-22pmol/L)
Thyroid-Stimulating Hormone	6.5mU/L (Ref: 0.27-4.2mU/L)
eGFR	>90mL/min/1.72m²
Prolactin	920mIU/L (100-850mIU/L)

What is the most likely diagnosis?
   a)   Thyrotrophinoma (TSHoma) with stalk compression
   b)   Sick Euthyroid Syndrome
   c)   Renal Failure
   d)   Hashimoto's Thyroiditis
   e)   Sleep-cycle disorder

#107. The catabolic pathway for producing thyroid hormones (T4 and T3) requires Iodide. Iodide, within the follicular cell must be transported across the apical surface to reach the follicular lumen, for which thyroid peroxidase converts iodide to iodine and attaches it to tyrosine residues on thyroglobulin. A deficiency of the transporter protein whose function is listed above leads to a peculiar constellation of symptoms, characterised by Hypothyroidism, Goitre, Congenital Sensorineural Hearing Loss, Vestibular Dysfunction and Temporal Bone Anomalies. Which of the following is the most likely diagnosis?
   a)   Pendred Syndrome
   b)   Pendrin Syndrome
   c)   Cretinism
   d)   Resistance to Thyroid Hormone Syndrome
   e)   Branchio-oto-renal Syndrome

#108. Which of the following is a causal factor for inadequate serum T4 despite optimal dosage of levothyroxine?
   a)   Inadequate storage of levothyroxine
   b)   Anti-thyroxine autoantibodies
   c)   Lactose-Intolerance
   d)   Recently converted from brand to generic medication
   e)   All of the above may be causal factors

#109. A 32-year-old gentleman presents to the family physician with the complaint of heat intolerance. After reviewing his past medical history, you note he is prescribed Zoloft; you consider this to be a side-effect of Zoloft and reduce the dosage with the patient's agreement. Six weeks later however, there is little improvement, and he is now describing the feeling of anxiety and impending doom most days of the week. Despite an increased appetite, he has noted to have lost around three kilograms in weight. His family history is unremarkable, with no thyroid disorders. A physical examination demonstrates a non-tender, normal-sized thyroid gland (no goitre), and gynaecomastia. Blood results are requested; however, the lab informs you there will be a turnover rate of two days. His past medical history is only significant for 'cryptoorchidism', for which at two years of age he underwent an orchiopexy to place the testicle within the scrotal sac. Which of the following is the likely cause of his symptoms?

    a)   Inadequate management of his anxiety
    b)   TSHoma
    c)   Atrophic Thyroiditis
    d)   Testicular Germ Cell Tumour
    e)   Phaeochromocytoma
    f)   None of the above

#110. The correct ratio of T4 to T3 requires the separate prescription of levothyroxine (T4) and Liothyronine (T3), as commercial preparations do not contain an adequate ratio. Which of the following is the recommended ratio of T4 to T3 to be prescribed in combination therapy?

    a)   5:1
    b)   15:1
    c)   1:1
    d)   1:5
    e)   1:15

#111. All of the following patients require an increase in the dosage of levothyroxine except for:

    a)   Growth Hormone Deficiency
    b)   Concurrent oral oestrogen
    c)   Concurrent Growth Hormone Replacement
    d)   High-dosage glucocorticoids
    e)   a) and d)

<u>#112.</u> For which of the following clinical situations will a dosage reduction of levothyroxine not be required:

    a)   Initiation of androgen therapy
    b)   Weight loss (above 10% of body weight)
    c)   Increasing age
    d)   Renal Failure
    e)   None of the above

<u>#113.</u> Infrequently, patients may demonstrate an allergic reaction to levothyroxine tablets; this is due to hypersensitivity to the dye or filler. Whilst dye sensitivity can be managed with white tablets, which of the following is the recommendation for sensitivity to fillers?

    a)   Parenteral administration
    b)   Soft-gel capsules
    c)   White tablets
    d)   All of the above are recommended

<u>#114.</u> Apart from a gluten-free diet, which of the following is a further recommendation to improve absorption of levothyroxine in patients with Coeliac's Disease?

    a)   Increasing the dosage
    b)   Parenteral administration
    c)   Once-weekly oral administration
    d)   Soft gel or liquid preparation
    e)   a) and d)

<u>#115.</u> A 66-year-old male with a carcinoma of the thyroid is scheduled to undergo a total thyroidectomy. The physician informs the patient he will require lifelong levothyroxine after the surgery. This patient should be told which of the following?

    a)   There is no residual thyroid tissue and thyroid hormones must be supplemented
    b)   Prevent recurrence of thyroid carcinoma by suppressing TSH
    c)   a) and b)
    d)   None of the above

<u>#116.</u> Liothyronine (T3) is seldom prescribed in clinical practice. For which of the following clinical situations is combination therapy appropriate?

    a)   Myxoedema Coma

b) DIO2 Gene mutation
c) Impaired quality of life with maximum levothyroxine replacement
d) b) and c)
e) a), b) and c)

#117. Glucocorticoids are prescribed in a myxoedema coma until adrenal insufficiency has been ruled out (to prevent an adrenal crisis). Which of the following best denotes the role of corticosteroids in a thyroid storm?

a) Glucocorticoids should not be prescribed in a thyroid storm
b) Glucocorticoids suppress the release of TSH, decreasing thyroid hormone release
c) Glucocorticoids inhibit the peripheral conversion of T4 to T3
d) b) and c)
e) a), b) and c)

#118. Which of the following medications is occasionally considered in a thyroid storm, functioning to decrease the enterohepatic circulation of thyroid hormones?

a) Cholic acid
b) Cholestyramine
c) Ezetimibe
d) Alirocumab
e) Niacin

#119. Tamoxifen is occasionally trialled for which of the following thyroid disorders?

a) DeQuervain's Thyroiditis
b) Riedel's Thyroiditis
c) Pyogenic Thyroiditis
d) Medullary Carcinoma
e) None of the above

#120. Which of the following are associated with an increased risk of developing autoimmune thyroid disease?

a) Noonan Syndrome
b) Trisomy 21
c) 45, XO

d) High Iodine Intake
e) b), c) and d)

#121. After initiation of a new dosage of levothyroxine, how long will it take for a steady state to be achieved?

a) Two weeks
b) Three weeks
c) Five weeks
d) Six weeks
e) Seven weeks

#122. Which of the following is **not** a complication of untreated hypothyroidism?

a) Hyperlipidaemia
b) Elevated serum creatine kinase
c) SIADH
d) Macrocytic Anaemia
e) Microcytic Anaemia
f) All of the above are complications

#123. Regarding the anatomy of the thyroid gland, which of the following is correct?

a) The left lobe is larger than the right lobe
b) The Pyramidal lobe may be present in at least one-third of people
c) The right lobe is larger than the left lobe
d) a) and b)
e) b) and c)

#124. Which of the following conditions of the thyroid gland may lead to amyloid deposition?

a) Papillary carcinoma
b) Medullary Thyroid carcinoma
c) Riedel's Thyroiditis
d) Hashimoto's Thyroiditis
e) None of the above

#125. Although medullary thyroid carcinoma is typically asymptomatic, occasionally calcitonin (and its gene products) may lead to all of the following except for:

a) Tetany

b) Diarrhoea
c) Pruritus
d) Flushing
e) None of the above

#126. An underlying pyriform sinus in a child may predispose to which of the following thyroid conditions?
a) DeQuervain's Thyroiditis
b) Riedel's Thyroiditis
c) Hashimoto's Thyroiditis
d) Pyogenic Thyroiditis
e) Tuberculosis of the thyroid gland

#127. A 26-year-old male with known Graves' Disease presents to his general practitioner. He is somewhat embarrassed and is reluctant to admit that since his diagnosis he was concerned he was growing breasts. Despite adherence to his daily carbimazole therapy, this has not resolved. Which of the following best explains how hyperthyroidism may lead to gynaecomastia?
a) Excess thyroid hormones increase the metabolism of androgens
b) Excess thyroid hormones increase the production of oestrogen
c) Hyperfunctioning thyroid tissue occasionally co-secretes oestrogen
d) Excess thyroid hormones increase the production of sex-hormone binding globulin (SHBG)
e) Gynaecomastia is not related to hyperthyroidism; consider exogenous steroid usage

#128. A 46-year-old female presents to her general practitioner with the complain of fatigue, malaise and menorrhagia, which has been ongoing for the last two years. Despite an active lifestyle and healthy dieting, she has gained around four kilograms in weight since the symptoms began around two years ago. Her medical history is insignificant apart from the occasional headache, which is related to her job as a secretary. Family history is furthermore non-contributory, apart from an uncle with atrial fibrillation. Upon physical examination, a goitre is palpable. The general practitioner requests the following investigations:

Free T4	14pmol/L (Ref: 12-22pmol/L)
Thyroid-Stimulating Hormone	7.0mU/L (Ref: 0.27-4.2mU/L)
Antithyroid Peroxidase	Positive ++
Haemoglobin (Hb)	15g/dL

What is the most likely diagnosis?

- a) Subclinical hyperthyroidism
- b) Assay interference
- c) Thyrotrophinoma
- d) Subclinical hypothyroidism
- e) Adrenal Insufficiency

#129. To confirm the diagnosis in question #128, a repeat TSH sample is recommended in three months' time (same time of day) to confirm the diagnosis, due to the variability of TSH (which returns unchanged at 7.0mU/L). Due to the presence of symptoms, she is commenced on 50 micrograms levothyroxine daily. Which of the following patients listed below do not require treatment with levothyroxine?

- a) 72-year-old asymptomatic gentleman with a TSH of 11.0mU/L with a medical history of a myocardial infarction five years prior
- b) 74-year-old female with a TSH of 10.5mU/L and profound hypothyroid symptomatology
- c) An asymptomatic 68-year-old male with a TSH of 7.0mU/L and a background history of bipolar disease
- d) A 44-year-old male with a TSH of 6.9mU/L and a palpable goitre
- e) a), b) and d)
- f) A 42-year-old female with a TSH of 7.2mU/L and recurrent of fatigue

#130. The thyroid gland and trachea are surrounded by a thin fascial layer. The posterior portion of the fascia adjoins the thyroid capsule, forming which of the following anatomical structures?

- a) Thyroidal Ligament
- b) Thyroid Ima Ligament
- c) Berry's Ligament
- d) Suspensory Ligament of the Thyroid Gland
- e) c) and d)

<u>#131</u>. An 11-year-old male is brought to his family physician by his mother. For the last six weeks he has been limping and refusing to bear weight on his left leg. There has been no recent trauma and he denies any recent upper respiratory tract infections. His past medical history includes mild intellectual impairment and hypothyroidism. On physical examination he is noted to be in the 10th centile for height but the 95th centile for weight. There is noticeable loss of external rotation of the hip. Which of the following is the most likely diagnosis?

    a)   Legg-Calve-Perthes Disease
    b)   Slipped Capital Femoral Epiphysis
    c)   Developmental Dysplasia of the Hip
    d)   Osteomalacia
    e)   Von-Recklinghausen's Disease of the Bone

<u>#132</u>. A 74-year-old gentleman with a background history of hypertension and atrial fibrillation is followed-up by his general practitioner. He is compliant with his polypharmacy of Warfarin, Bisoprolol and Ramipril, however there is little improvement. Within the clinic, his blood pressure remains above 150/90mmHg, and an irregularly-irregular pulse is identified by the nurse. Although he is asymptomatic, the physician the following laboratory investigations:

Free T4	16pmol/L (Ref: 12-22pmol/L)
Thyroid-Stimulating Hormone	<0.01mU/L (Ref: 0.27-4.2mU/L)

Which of the following is the most likely diagnosis?

    a)   Sick Euthyroid Syndrome
    b)   Subclinical hypothyroidism
    c)   TSH suppression by medication
    d)   Falsely elevated free T4 by medication
    e)   Subclinical hyperthyroidism

<u>#133.</u> Which of the following is a sentinel lymph node for which is removed during a total thyroidectomy, to determine metastatic spread?

    a)   Delphian Lymph Node
    b)   Infraclavicular
    c)   Submandibular
    d)   Sublingual
    e)   All of the above

#134. The recurrent laryngeal nerve medially to which of the following anatomical landmarks used in head and neck surgery?
  a)   Pyramidal Lobe
  b)   Thyroglossal Duct
  c)   Torus Tubarius
  d)   Torus Palatinus
  e)   Tubercle of Zuckerkandl

#135. The thyroid gland receives its blood supply from the superior and inferior thyroid arteries. Occasionally however, an embryonic (third) artery may be present, known as the thyroid artery of Neubauer (Thyroid Ima Artery). From which of the following structures does this artery most commonly arise from?
  a)   Right subclavian artery
  b)   Brachiocephalic trunk
  c)   Left carotid artery
  d)   Inferior thyroid artery
  e)   Thyrocervical trunk

#136. Apart from a thyrotrophinoma (TSHoma) of the pituitary gland, which of the following pituitary disorders can present with a goitre?
  a)   Cushing's Disease
  b)   Prolactinoma
  c)   Sheehan's Syndrome
  d)   Acromegaly
  e)   All of the above

#137. Autoimmune hypothyroidism is more common than secondary hypothyroidism (hypopituitarism). Diagnostic dilemma arises as patients with hypothyroidism may present with hyperprolactinaemia and an adenoma of the pituitary gland (misdiagnosed as a macroprolactinoma with mass compression of the thyrotrophes). Apart from an incidentaloma, which of the following is the most likely explanation for a pituitary adenoma in long-standing, untreated hypothyroidism?
  a)   Concurrent prolactinoma
  b)   Metastases
  c)   Hashimoto's Encephalopathy
  d)   Artefact
  e)   Thyrotrophe Hyperplasia

#138. A mother brings her 6-year-old daughter to the paediatric endocrinologist, in order to answer some queries. The girl has been diagnosed with hypothyroidism six months ago and has been managed with levothyroxine. The mother has read a recent article in the newspaper stating 'thyroid disorders may lead to premature puberty'; it did not say if this was due to hypothyroidism or hyperthyroidism, and she would like to know if her daughter will develop precocious puberty (and hence shorter final stature). Which of the following is the correct response?

a) Hyperthyroidism may lead to precocious puberty; this is known as van-Wyck-Grumbach Syndrome
b) Hypothyroidism may lead to delayed puberty; this is known as van-Wyck-Grumbach Syndrome
c) Hypothyroidism can lead to precocious puberty; when associated with ovarian cysts, this is known as van-Wyck-Grumbach Syndrome
d) Hyperthyroidism can lead to precocious puberty; when associated with ovarian cysts, this is known as van-Wyck-Grumbach Syndrome
e) There is no association between thyroid disorders and altered onset of puberty

#139. Which of the following lysosomal storage disorders can present with hypothyroidism as a consequence in untreated patients?

a) Homocystinuria
b) Cystinosis
c) Hyperoxaluria
d) Trimethylaminuria
e) Cystinuria

#140. A certain medication is used in the management of multiple myeloma, however, is best known for its teratogenic effects, with infants born with phocomelia. This medication has also been known to occasionally lead to hypothyroidism. Which of the following options is the medication described?

a) Voriconazole
b) Amphotericin
c) Thalidomide
d) Bortezomib
e) Propylthiouracil

#141. Multiple Endocrine Neoplasia Type 2A may present with 'the two M's and one P' (i.e., medullary thyroid carcinoma, parathyroid hyperplasia and phaeochromocytoma). Which of the following lesions may also be present in the thyroid gland and must be considered as a differential diagnosis to medullary thyroid carcinoma?

a) Metastasis
b) Paraganglioma
c) Lymphoma
d) All of the above
e) None of the above

#142. Which of the following underlying haematological disorders may interfere with thyroid hormone assays, presenting with either spurious T3 toxicosis or elevated TSH?

a) Macrocytic, Megaloblastic Anaemia
b) Microcytic, Normochromic Anaemia
c) Sideroblastic Anaemia
d) Multiple Myeloma
e) Paroxysmal Nocturnal Haemaglobinuria

#143. A 38-year-old female with a past medical history of illness-anxiety disorder attends her family physician. Her best friend of 20 years has recently been diagnosed with tracheal cancer, and she is very concerned she could have it as well. Despite the absence of a smoking history, she cannot put her mind at ease. She thinks she may have felt a lump in her neck but is unsure if her mind is playing tricks on her. Her family physician performs a full neck examination and does not palpate any abnormality. The patient requests if she could have a thyroid hormone panel, as her sister suffers from Graves' Disease, and this would put her mind at ease. After much argument, the physician agrees (if the patient attends cognitive-behavioural-therapy sessions). The following blood results return:

Free T4	25pmol/L (Ref: 12-22pmol/L)
Thyroid-Stimulating Hormone	2.2mU/L (Ref: 0.27-4.2mU/L)

Which of the following is the next best step?

a) TSH Receptor Autoantibody titre
b) Anti-thyroid peroxidase titre
c) Reassurance
d) Commence carbimazole
e) Commence propranolol

<u>#144.</u> With reference to question #143, which of the following is the underlying diagnosis?

- a) Hashitoxicosis
- b) Assay interference
- c) Factitious Thyrotoxicosis
- d) Palpation Thyroiditis
- e) Thyroid Carcinoma

<u>#145.</u> In the 1970s in North America, the fast-food industries began to expand throughout the major cities. Many patients noted to eat from the fast-food restaurants however, developed hyperactive symptoms, for which led to an initial conclusion preservatives in the food may lead to ADHD. This was later disproved however, when these patients were found to display elevated serum free T3 and T4 levels. This became known as 'Hamburger Thyrotoxicosis'. Which of the following is the underlying causative factor?

- a) Thyroid hormone supplemented to the cattle
- b) Inadequate refrigeration
- c) Ingestion of Thyroid tissue
- d) Thyroid supplements added to uncooked meat
- e) All of the above

<u>#146.</u> After diagnosing a 33-year-old kindergarten teacher with Graves' Disease, she is commenced upon carbimazole therapy and is followed up in six weeks' time for necessary dosage adjustments. Her results at diagnosis and at follow-up are demonstrated below.

	At Diagnosis	Six-Week Follow-Up
Free T4	26pmol/L (Ref: 12-22pmol/L)	21pmol/L (Ref: 12-22pmol/L)
TSH	<0.01mU/L (Ref: 0.27-4.2mU/L)	<0.01mU/L (Ref: 0.27-4.2mU/L)

The visiting medical student is concerned about the low TSH at follow-up, and asks if this suggests a poor response? Which of the following is the correct response?

- a) After treatment, a low TSH at follow-up suggests likely resistance to the medication
- b) TSH is not used to monitor treatment
- c) After treatment, a low TSH at follow-up suggests likely sensitivity to the medication
- d) TSH is not used in the first few month's post-initiation of medication
- e) None of the above

#147. Hashimoto's Thyroiditis is the best-known cause of autoimmune hypothyroidism in the developed world. Hashimoto's thyroiditis may lead to a goitre, transient hyperthyroid state and hypothyroidism from lymphocytic infiltration. Another form of thyroiditis, known as Ord's Thyroiditis, is further caused by autoantibodies directed towards the thyroid gland. Which of the following options best distinguishes the two clinical disorders?

- a) Ord's Thyroiditis presents with a more prominent goitre
- b) Ord's Thyroiditis presents with atrophy, not goitre
- c) Ord's Thyroiditis presents without a transient hyperthyroid phase
- d) a) and c)
- e) b) and c)

#148. A 24-year-old female is commenced upon Epoprostenol for primary pulmonary hypertension. She has a positive family history, for which her mother unfortunately developed acute cor pulmonale. Which of the following must she be warned about prior to commencing Epoprostenol?

- a) Goitrogen
- b) Thyroid Tissue Pigmentation
- c) Hypothyroidism
- d) Hyperthyroidism
- e) Carcinogenic

#149. A medical student asks you what the difference is between hyperthyroidism and thyrotoxicosis. How do you response?

- a) The terms are interchangeable
- b) Thyrotoxicosis refers to an hyperfunctioning thyroid gland
- c) Hyperthyroidism is an umbrella term to refer to the phenotype of hyper-functional thyroid tissue
- d) Hyperthyroidism refers to hyperfunctioning thyroid tissue whereas thyrotoxicosis refers to the clinical phenotype
- e) b) and c)

#150. Cranial Synostosis is a foetal complication of which of the following?

a) Carbimazole exposure
b) Uncontrolled hypothyroidism in-utero
c) Propylthiouracil exposure
d) Uncontrolled hyperthyroidism in-utero
e) Cretinism

#151. Thyroid cancer is very unlikely to ever be 'active', however rare case reports have documented which of the following metastatic thyroid cancers to release hormones and contribute to hyperthyroidism?

a) Hashimoto's Lymphoma
b) Papillary Carcinoma
c) Follicular Carcinoma
d) Anaplastic Carcinoma
e) Medullary Thyroid Carcinoma

#152. Which of the following are dietary goitrogens?

a) Vitamin A
b) Selenium
c) Cabbage, Cauliflower, Broccoli
d) Iron
e) a) and c)

#153. Bexarotene, an antineoplastic medication used in the management for T-cell lymphoma (Mycosis Fungoides) may lead to which of the following endocrine complications?

a) Hashimoto's Thyroiditis
b) Graves' Disease
c) Central Hypothyroidism
d) Drug-Induced Thyroiditis
e) Follicular Carcinoma

#154. Which of the following options best characterises the following description: Intellectual Disability, Deaf, Mutism, Gait Disturbance and Spasticity, but **no hypothyroidism.**

a) Neurologic Cretinism
b) Myxoedematous Cretinism
c) Hashimoto's Encephalopathy
d) Myxoedema Coma

#155. Fine-needle aspiration cytology is reliable for all types of thyroid cancer, except for which of the following?

a) Papillary
b) Follicular
c) Medullary
d) Anaplastic
e) None of the above

#156. Which of the following best matches a thyroid disorder and its corresponding effect upon the vasculature system?

a) Hyperthyroidism; Hypotension
b) Hypothyroidism; Hypotension
c) Hyperthyroidism; Diastolic Hypertension
d) Hypothyroidism; Systolic Hypertension
e) Hyperthyroidism; Systolic Hypertension

#157. A 62-year-male is transferred to the emergency department with the complaint of 'pins and needles' around both his ankles and feet. A physical examination performed demonstrates weakness with both dorsiflexion and plantarflexion. He has a past medical history of hypothyroidism diagnosed two years ago and is currently under investigation for multiple myeloma. Moreover, an abdominal examination reveals dullness to percussion in Traube's space (splenomegaly) and a tanned appearance. Which of the following is the most likely diagnosis?

a) Haemochromatosis
b) Wilson's Disease
c) Multiple Myeloma
d) POEMS Syndrome
e) Amyloidosis

#158. The association with thyroid disease and ANCA+ vasculitis is:

a) The presence of one autoimmune condition predisposes the risk to acquiring another
b) Thionamide medications used in the management of hyperthyroidism may cause ANCA positive vasculitis
c) Levothyroxine used in the treatment of hypothyroidism may cause ANCA positive vasculitis
d) All of the above

<u>#159.</u> After an unremarkably pregnancy, a 32-year-old mother with Graves' Disease would like to know if she can breastfeed. Which of the following is the correct response?

a) Patients with Graves' Disease should not breastfeed, due to the transfer of autoantibodies in the milk
b) Patients can only breastfeed if thionamide medications are stopped, as they appear in the breast milk
c) Patients can breastfeed only on propylthiouracil, not carbimazole
d) Patients can breastfeed only on carbimazole, not propylthiouracil
e) Patients can breastfeed on either medication

<u>#160.</u> A 32-year-old female has been hospitalised with severe streptococcal pneumonia, requiring ITU care. For reasons that are unclear, the junior doctor decides to order a thyroid hormone profile, demonstrated below. Although concerned, the consultant dismisses this as 'Sick Euthyroid Syndrome'. After two-weeks in hospital the patient has recovered with little sequelae apart from tiredness. The junior doctor orders a repeat thyroid hormone profile prior to her discharge, demonstrated below:

	On Admission	Prior to Discharge
Free T4	10pmol/L (Ref: 12-22pmol/L)	18pmol/L (Ref: 12-22pmol/L)
TSH	0.20mU/L (Ref: 0.27-4.2mU/L)	4.6mU/L (Ref: 0.27-4.2mU/L)

Which of the following is the likely explanation for elevated TSH?

a) Subclinical hypothyroidism
b) Thyrotrophinoma
c) Recovery from Sick Euthyroid Syndrome
d) Recurrent Sick Euthyroid Syndrome
e) MacroTSH

Thyroid Gland – Answers

<u>#1.</u> b) Medication Interaction
Patients may not include over-the-counter medications in their list they provide to their physicians. It is vital to specifically ask if they are taking anything over-the-counter due to the potential for medication interactions. In this case, with a past medical history of fibroids, it is very likely that this patient has been taking iron tablets (such as ferrous sulphate), which can be purchased over the counter. All patients must be advised to take Levothyroxine on an empty stomach (first thing in the morning), with all other medications (and food) at least an hour later. Ferrous sulphate (as well as many other medications) interferes with the absorption of Levothyroxine, and therefore despite her compliance in this case study, there is malabsorption. Non-compliance is always a potential concern; patients may take their levothyroxine prior to the blood test, in which case a demonstration of increased free T4 and inadequate TSH will be present.

<u>#2.</u> b) Vitamin B7
Biotin (Vitamin B7) must be withheld 48 hours prior to a thyroid hormone panel, as it may interfere with the assay, leading to falsely elevated free T4 and falsely suppressed TSH. Moreover, a false-increase in serum titre of autoantibodies may be demonstrated.

<u>#3.</u> b) Thyroid Function Tests
In addition to nephrogenic diabetes insipidus, Lithium is known to induce hypothyroidism, which requires long-term follow up of the thyroid function tests. Moreover, Lithium may cause a goitre in up to 50% of patients (with or without hypothyroidism). Although Lithium may lead to hyperparathyroidism, this is much less common than Lithium-induced hypothyroidism.

<u>#4.</u> e) 150 micrograms
The World Health Organization recommend for non-pregnant healthy adults to intake 150 micrograms of iodine per day. In lactating or pregnant women, this is increased to 200 micrograms. Moreover, in children, between 50 to 250 micrograms are recommended. Urinary 24-hour iodine collection can be used to estimate dietary intake as iodine is excreted by the renal system (30-50mL/minute).

#5. c) and d) (option e)
Thyroglobulin is used to screen for recurrence after treatment for papillary thyroid carcinoma (not medullary thyroid carcinoma). It is inappropriate to use serum thyroglobulin levels as a marker for cancer, only for monitoring. Thyroglobulin is also used as an integral part of the diagnosis for factitious hyperthyroidism, whereby levels are decreased (as opposed to thyroiditis, where the levels are increased). One must be wary however, as in the presence of antithyroglobulin autoantibodies (autoimmune thyroid disease), the assay may lead to falsely lowered thyroglobulin levels.

#6. c) 80% is produced by the deiodinase enzymatic system in the periphery
The thyroid gland is responsible for only 20% of circulating T3; 80% is produced as a result of peripheral conversion from T4 to T3 through the enzymatic system deiodinase. Three types (D1, D2 and D3) are present, with D2 contributing to the majority of extrathyroidal T3 production.

#7. e) Normal gestational phenomenon
Excess beta-hCG in pregnancy may bind to the TSH receptors and can cause negative feedback resulting in lowered TSH. Additionally, oestrogen promotes the synthesis of thyroxine-binding globulin (TBG), leading to an increased total T4 level, however the free T4 level is unchanged. The nausea and vomiting are normal for morning sickness in the first trimester, with her occasional headaches likely a recurrence of her migraines. This patient does not have Graves' Disease.

#8. b) and d) (option e)
The diagnosis is of a thyroglossal duct cyst. This is harmless, and is typically operated upon for cosmetic reasons, for which the procedure is a sistrunk operation. He is asymptomatic and the location and character of the lesion are not typical for leukaemia; moreover, thyroglossal duct cysts are associated with normal underlying thyroid tissue.

#9. c) In the presence of a sore throat or fever, discontinue the medication and seek urgent medical attention
An uncommon (but fatal) side effect of thionamide medications may be agranulocytosis. In the setting of a sore throat or fever, these patients must discontinue the medications and seek urgent medical

attention. Although teratogenic effects can occur, these medications can be continued during pregnancy. Moreover, drug-induced vasculitis (ANCA positivity) may occur with commencement of the drug (and disappear with discontinuation of the medication). Only carbimazole is a pro-drug.

#10. a) Amiodarone
Amiodarone is composed of iodine (37% of its weight) and therefore in iodine-deficient patients, may promote hyperthyroidism. In iodine-sufficient patients, may promote hypothyroidism.

#11. d) Levothyroxine must be continued, but at an increased dose
Levothyroxine is essential as this will be the only supply of thyroid hormone to the foetus in the first trimester of pregnancy. The mother will therefore need to increase the dosage by around 50%. Liothyronine (T3) must never be commenced when pregnant, as it is teratogenic.

#12. c) Foramen Caecum
The Thyroid gland beings its development at the Foramen Caecum, located on the lingual tissue between the tuberculum impar and copula.

#13. d) Fourth Pharyngeal Pouch
The Fourth Pharyngeal Pouch gives rise to the C-cells of the thyroid gland, in addition to the superior parathyroid gland.

#14. d) Medullary Thyroid Carcinoma
This patient's family history is suggestive of Multiple Endocrine Neoplasia, Type 2A, characterised by Hyperparathyroidism (not from a carcinoma), Phaeochromocytoma and Medullary Thyroid Carcinoma.

#15. b) Heterophile Antibody Interference
This vignette hints that she is around animals, which may interfere with thyroid assays falsely suggesting elevated TSH. Assay interference is much more common than a true TSHoma (thyrotrophinoma).

#16. a) Medullary Thyroid Carcinoma
Calcitonin can be used as a tumour marker for recurrence of (not diagnosis of) Medullary Thyroid Carcinoma. Additionally, CEA may be elevated, which can be managed with anti-CEA autoantibodies.

<u>**#17.**</u> d) Smoking
Smoking is the strongest risk factor for the development (and relapse) of both Graves' Disease and Graves' Ophthalmopathy. Smoking cessation is the single most important aspect of management.

<u>**#18.**</u> c) Yersinia Enterocolitica
Yersinia is known to contain TSH binding sites, with autoantibodies to Yersinia noted to be present in patients with Graves' Disease. Titres are seen at higher levels in identical twins (one of which demonstrates Graves' Disease) compared to Dizygotic Twins.

<u>**#19.**</u> d) Struma Ovarii
Teratomas of the ovary, which are more common amongst younger adult females, may occasionally contain ectopic thyroid tissue. As with this patient ovarian tumours may present with non-specific abdominal signs such as 'bloating'. The Sturma Ovarii releases thyroid hormones, with negative feedback leading to suppression of TSH release (and therefore absence of goitre/thyroid atrophy).

<u>**#20.**</u> b) Aplasia Cutis; Carbimazole
Carbimazole (or Methimazole) is known to harbour teratogenic effects in pregnancy and is therefore only used after the first trimester. One of the potential complications from Carbimazole is Aplasia Cutis of the newborn.

<u>**#21.**</u> e) All of the above
Signs specific to Graves' Disease include Thyroid Acropachy, Thyroid Bruit, Pretibial Myxoedema and hyperpigmentation of the upper eyelid (Jellinek's Sign) (amongst many others).

Eponymous Sign	Description
Abadie's Sign	Spastic Levator muscle of upper eyelid
Ballett's Sign	Pupil and automatic reactions are preserved, with abolishment too voluntary movements
Boston's Sign	Spasticity of Levator upon downward gaze - faster closure of eyelid
Beck's Sign	Intense pulsation of retinal arteries when viewing fundus
Cowen's Sign	Pupillary constriction is exaggerated and rapid (internal musculature involvement)
Darlymple's Sign	**Commonest Sign:** Iris inappropriately discovered from eyelids (widened palpebral fissure)
Enroth's Sign	Lower lid oedema
Gifford's Sign	Retracted upper eyelid yields difficulty in eversion

Griffith Sign	Lower lid lag on downward gaze
Goldzieher's Sign	Deep injection of conjunctiva at site of insertion of extra ocular muscles
Grove's Sign	Resistance on upper lid (retracted) being pulled down
Hertoghe Sign	Eyebrow's lost in outer 1/3 of eyelid (also known as Queen Anne's Sign; more likely in Hypothyroidism)
Jellinek's Sign	Superior eye-fold hyper pigmentation
Jendrassik's Sign	Restricted abduction and rotation of globe
Joffroy's Sign	Superior gaze is associated with absence of creases on forehead
Knie's Sign	Dim light is associated with unequal dilatation of pupils
Kocher's Sign	Staring (visual fixation) leads to increased lid retraction
Loewi's Sign	Mydriasis is rapid upon low concentration of epinephrine
Mann's Sign	Tanned appearance of skin suggests eyes appear at different levels
Möbius' Sign	Difficulty/inability with convergence
Movement Cap Phenomenon	Movements of globe are incomplete, abrupt and with difficulty
Payne-Trouseau's Sign	Globe luxation (dislocation)
Pochin's Sign	Decreased amplitude of blinking
Rosenbach's Sign	Closed eyelids demonstrated tremor
Russel-Fraser's Sign	Fold between eyeball and upper eyelid narrowed upon closure of eyes
Sainton's Sign	Forehead wrinkling is delayed with up gaze
Sattler's Sign	Upgaze leads to increased intraocular pressure
Snellen-Riesman's Sign	Bruit over closed eye (during systole) with stethoscope for auscultation
Stellwag's Sign	Infrequent blinking (looks as if patient is staring)
Suker's Sign	Improper fixation with abduction
Tella's Sign	Hyperpigmentation of inferior eyelid
Topolanski's Sign	Vascular network donated around rectus muscle (x4) insertion points
Vigoroux's Sign	Swelling of eyelid (fullness)
von Graefe's Sign	Downward gaze is associated with lid-lag of upper eyelid
Willibrand-Saenger's Sign	Increased drip secretion to protect from lagophthalmos
Wilder's Sign	Abduction to adduction leads to rapid jerking of the eye

#22. c) Selenium

Selenium is recommended as first-line for mild (active) Graves' Ophthalmopathy.

#23. c) Superior Thyroid Artery (branch of External Carotid Artery) and Inferior Thyroid Artery (branch of Subclavian Artery)

The superior thyroid artery is a branch of the external carotid artery, with the inferior thyroid artery a branch of the subclavian artery. Moreover, the venous drainage is from three veins: Superior and Middle Thyroid Veins (draining into Internal Jugular Vein) and the Inferior Thyroid Vein (draining into the Left Brachiocephalic Vein).

#24. c) T3

This is a case of clear hyperthyroidism despite normal serum free T4. The diagnosis in this case is T3 Toxicosis, which is responsible for up to 5% of cases of hyperthyroidism.

#25. d) Hypokalaemic (Thyrotoxic) Periodic Paralysis

This is a neuromuscular disorder characterised by muscular weakness (painless) induced by fasting, heavy exercise or carbohydrate-heavy meals. It typically is inherited as either an autosomal dominant disorder or acquired from thyrotoxicosis, most prevalent in Asian populations. The great majority of patients demonstrate a mutation in the SCN4A skeletal muscle sodium channel.

#26. a) and c) (option d)

Hashimoto's Thyroiditis is known to increase the risk of Lymphoma, Papillary Carcinoma, Hashimoto's Encephalopathy and other Autoimmune Disorders.

#27. c) 12-18 months

Hyperthyroid patients are typically treated with thionamide medications for 12-18 months, at which the autoantibody titres are measured, and the physician may consider withdrawing (and ultimately stopping) the medication.

#28. b) The GREAT Score

The GREAT (Graves' Recurrent Events after Therapy) Score has been validated to assess the risk of relapse for Graves' Disease after therapy.

#29. b) Hepatitis C

There is a higher prevalence of autoantibodies towards Hepatitis C in patients with Hashimoto's thyroiditis compared to normal cohorts.

#30. b) Beta-blockers
Beta-blockers are typically initiated first when a patient has symptomatic hyperthyroidism, to decrease palpitations, tremor and act as an anxiolytic.

#31. d) Administration of iodine inhibits thyroid hormone release
The ingestion of large amounts of iodine promotes inhibition of organification within the thyroid gland, with decreased thyroid hormone synthesis and release. The Wolff-Chaikoff effect is best demonstrated with the example of a thyroid storm.

#32. c) Tachycardia
The Meresburg Triad is the constellation of Exophthalmos, Goitre and Palpitations (Tachycardia), suggestive of Graves' Disease.

#33. c) and d) (option e)
HLA-DR3 and CTLA-4 are known associates with the development of Graves' Disease within the Caucasian population.

#34. b) and c) (option e)
The Medial Rectus and Inferior Rectus are most severely affected in Graves' Ophthalmopathy

#35. a) HLA-DRB107
Patients harbouring the HLA-DRB107 haplotype (for reasons unknown) demonstrate a reduced risk of acquiring Graves' Disease.

 #36. c) NOSPECS
The NOSPECS Scoring System allows classification of Thyroid Eye Disease; NOSPECS is a mnemonic for:

      No signs/symptoms
      Only signs
      Soft tissue is involved (with symptoms and signs)
      Proptosis
      Extraocular muscular involvement
      Cornea is involved
      Sight loss

#37. b) Vitamin D
Low levels of Vitamin D are more frequently identified in patients with Graves' Disease; it is unclear if this is cause-or-effect, however, many

autoimmune disorders (such as SLE, Multiple Sclerosis) note a similar finding.

#38. b) Pre-treatment with thionamides
Thionamides are used to reduce the risk of thyroiditis and/or thyroid storm post-ablation. Medications are typically initiated at least one month prior to the procedure and withdrawn four days before the ablation (and recommenced four days after the procedure). Patients must not be pregnant, must not be around children, nor can there be thyroid cancer. Severe Grave's Ophthalmopathy may be exacerbated by radioiodine treatment; although concurrent treatment with glucocorticoids may be possible, other treatment options may be more appropriate.

#39. d) Pre-treatment with propylthiouracil
All of the listed options have successfully been used to decrease the risk of post-ablative thyroiditis and/or thyroid storm, however, propylthiouracil is best known for a decreased effectiveness compared to carbimazole.

#40. e) All of the above
A thyroidectomy will result in permanent hypothyroidism. Moreover, the parathyroid glands may be removed in a total thyroidectomy, leading to hypocalcaemia. Local structures such as the recurrent and superior laryngeal nerves are at risk of transection. Depending on the clinical situation, without adequate pre-operative treatment, a thyroid storm may be precipitated. Finally, post-surgery there is a risk for wound haematoma formation – for this reason a scalpel is kept near the bedside to be able to open the wound and prevent airway compression in the presence of suspicion of an expanding haematoma.

#41. c) Six Months
Females with graves' disease desiring pregnancy in whom medications are not appropriate should be treated with radioablation or total thyroidectomy; it is universally agreed upon to have this done at least six months prior to attempts to conceive.

#42. a) IgG
IgG is the only antibody to cross the placenta and hence may cause transient neonatal thyrotoxicosis in infants born to a mother with Graves' Disease.

#43. b) Carbimazole
This case vignette is demonstrative of Choanal Atresia, a rare teratogenic effect of Carbimazole.

#44. b) Jod-Basedow Phenomenon
This is the 'opposite' of the Wolff-Chaikoff effect, whereby excess iodine administration in iodine-deficient patients may promote thyrotoxicosis.

#45. c) Anti-insulin antibodies (hypoglycaemia)
Hirata's Syndrome is a very uncommon condition with less than one-hundred cases described in the literature. Most prevalent amongst Japanese individuals, this disorder is noted by the association of Graves' Disease, Carbimazole and anti-insulin autoantibodies, with resultant hypoglycaemia.

#46. e) Propylthiouracil
A teratogenic effect of propylthiouracil (although extremely uncommon) is the development of Situs Inversus.

#47. a) and b) (option e)
This vignette describes a patient with a retrosternal goitre (noted by the dullness to percussion amongst the anterior sternum and Pemberton's Sign). The retrosternal goitre has led to compression of the superior vena cava, producing venous distension and engorgement of upper limbs and face.

#48. b) Thyroid Storm
This patient demonstrates a thyroid storm, a clinical emergency requiring prompt treatment.

#49. c) Burch and Wartofsky
The Burch and Wartofsky Point Scale (1993) is a scoring system for a thyroid storm. A score of 45 or more is suggestive of a thyroid storm, whereby under 25 a thyroid storm is highly unlikely. A score of between 25 and 44 may suggest an 'impending thyroid storm'.

#50. d) Androgens
Androgens are known to decrease Thyroxine-Binding Globulin (TBG), whereas the other options are known to increase TBG.

#51. b) ESR (Westergren)
Symptoms of DeQuervain's Thyroiditis include dysphagia, tenderness upon palpation and a low-grade fever. The condition occurs a couple weeks after an upper respiratory tract infection (including COVID-19) and is a result of transient thyrotoxicosis due to the release of preformed hormones. Although this is difficult at times to differentiate from Grave's Disease, the ESR (Westergren) will be massively elevated with DeQuervain's Thyroiditis.

#52. d) Thyroid Hormone Resistance Syndrome
The case vignette is describing Thyroid Hormone Resistance Syndrome, alternatively referred to as Refetoff Syndrome. This condition is denoted by an impaired sensitivity (either within the pituitary or peripherally) to thyroid hormones, therefore there is elevation of the TSH to overcome this reduced sensitivity. The underlying cause in greater than 80% of patients is due to the beta-subtype of the thyroid hormone receptor on chromosome three, occurring de novo or as autosomal dominant inheritance. Symptoms will vary between individuals of the same genetic mutation as a result of differentiation of tissue sensitivity to thyroid hormones. Symptoms may include goitre, ENT infections, sensorineural hearing loss, learning disabilities, ADHD-type behaviour and tachycardia. This is differentiated from a pituitary tumour (TSHoma), whereby the levels of TSH increase in response to TRH with Refetoff Syndrome (and not with a TSHoma).

#53. b) Heterophile Antibody Interference
Heterophile Antibody Interference is much more common than a true 'TSHoma' and hence must always be assessed for in the history before requesting an MRI scan of the pituitary; it is important to note up to 10% of the population may demonstrate a pituitary incidentaloma and this may erroneously be diagnosed as a TSHoma without a proper history.

#54. d) Familial Dysalbuminaemic Hyperthyroxinaemia
This is an autosomal dominant disorder characterised by a mutation in albumin molecules, leading to lower affinity (but higher capacity) for T4 (not T3). Total T4 is increased however free T4 is relatively unaltered as is TSH; these patients require no treatment.

#55. c) Alpha Subunit
The alpha subunit of TSH may be elevated in the serum of patients with a TSHoma, but not those with Thyroid Hormone Resistance Syndrome.

#56. b) Drug-induced Graves' Disease
Alemtuzumab is a monoclonal antibody directed towards CD52, used in the treatment of Multiple Sclerosis. A peculiar side effect of this medication is the increase frequency of patients administered Alemtuzumab developing Graves' Disease; Alemtuzumab-induced Graves' Disease has a high remission rate.

#57. c) Minocycline
Minocycline, a tetracycline antibiotic most commonly used in the treatment of acne vulgaris, is known to cause black pigmentation of the thyroid gland. Moreover, at low doses, minocycline acts as a competitive inhibitor of Thyroid Peroxidase iodination (thyroid disease, however, is extremely unlikely).

#58. c) Metformin Administration
All of the listed options are known to increase TSH serum levels, except for Metformin, for which patients administered are more likely to demonstrate decreased levels.

#59. a) Multinodular Goitre
Multinodular Goitres are the second most common cause of Hyperthyroidism and are more prevalent amongst the elderly population. It is vital to rule out this diagnosis as the management options will vary depending on the underlying cause – unlikely to be cured with thionamides and are best treated with radioablation or surgery.

#60. e) Macro-TSH
Medications may decrease the levels of TSH by means of direct receptor action, or from Hypophysitis (Checkpoint inhibitors). Afro-caribbeans are known to harbour decreased (but still normal) levels of TSH. All other options listed may decrease levels of TSH, apart from 'Macro-TSH'. This is a laboratory artefact whereby TSH and immunoglobulins form a macromolecule, spuriously increasing the measured TSH levels. This should always be considered as a differential

diagnosis to subclinical hypothyroidism. MacroTSH may be confirmed by gel filtration chromatography.

#61. b) Decreased Free T4
Antiepileptic medications such as phenytoin may increase the metabolism of free T4, leading to spuriously lowered levels on measurement.

#62. b) and d) (option e)
Via incompletely understood mechanisms, heparin activates lipoprotein lipase, which increases free fatty acids. These prevent the binding of thyroxine to albumin and TBG.

#63. d) Aspirin; Prednisone
A stepwise approach is recommended in managing the inflammation/neck discomfort in DeQuervain's Thyroidits. Patients should begin with non-steroidal-anti-inflammatory drugs (such as aspirin) when discomfort and systemic symptoms are mild. If there is no improvement in three days (or if symptoms are severe), NSAIDs are discontinued, and Prednisone is initiated.

#64. b) HLA-B35
HLA-B35 is associated with the development of DeQuervain's Thyroiditis.

#65. c) Lymphocytic Hypophysitis
Lymphocytic Hypophysitis is a rare endocrine disorder characterised by lymphocytic infiltration and fibrosis of the pituitary gland. This is most common in patients towards the end of pregnancy, or post-partum. A characteristic radiological sign of Lymphocytic Hypophysitis is 'stalk enhancement'. Moreover, Lymphocytic Hypophysitis may demonstrate 'isolated TSH deficiency'. Although this may be difficult to distinguish from Sheehan's Syndrome, the normal levels of IGF-1 in the serum rule out against pituitary infarction (Growth Hormone would be the first hormone affected in hypopituitarism, suggesting the deficiency is limited to TSH).

#66. c) Non-compliance (Pseudomalabsorption)
The most common cause of persistently deranged thyroid function tests would be non-compliance (pseudomalabsorption). Other causes are considered once compliance is established.

#67. a) Anti-tissue transglutaminase antibody

The vignette demonstrates a patient undergoing the T4-absorption test. After a large dosage administered (and supervised) orally, there is suboptimal serum T4 with repeat samples. This suggests malabsorption; the patient has autoimmune thyroiditis and there is a family history of type 1 diabetes mellitus. One must consider a further autoimmune condition for this patient, for which Coeliac's Disease is the likely culprit. The prevalence of Coeliac's Disease is 5% amongst patients with autoimmune hypothyroidism compared to 1% of the general population. Many patients (as in this case study) do not demonstrate symptoms, and the diagnosis is only confirmed with histological samples or autoantibody titres.

#68. c) Once-weekly oral ingestion

For patients with poor adherence to daily thyroxine, the American Thyroid Association recommend once-weekly oral ingestion. The evidence for this however, involves limited trials of a few years' follow-up, for which the long-term effects are unknown. In the short-term, it does appear to be safe, however, the limited data is only available for oral (and not parenteral) administration. Dosages between 1,000 and 1,500 micrograms may be administered, with little increased side-effects noted.

#69. c) and d) (option e)

Levothyroxine may worsen angina and atrial fibrillation, therefore cautious up-titration is recommended in elderly patients.

#70. b) Pregnancy

Combination therapy is contraindicated in pregnancy, as foetal neurological development is dependent upon the maternal free T4 concentrations until up to 18 weeks' gestation; administration of T3 has led to slightly decreased T4 levels and limited anecdotes have demonstrated impaired neurological development by induction of hypothyroxinaemia.

#71. a) Consumptive Hypothyroidism

Consumptive Hypothyroidism is a rare disorder characterised by cutaneous and liver haemangiomas. Within the haemangiomas, there is increased production of the type 3 Deiodinase Enzyme (D3), which degrades both T4 and T3 into metabolites which are inactive, with resultant increased reverse T3.

#72. c) Iodine accumulation
The kidneys are involved in the excretion of iodide, therefore with a decrease in eGFR, the iodide accumulates and may be added to the thyroid pool. Increase iodide may block thyroid hormone synthesis by way of the Wolff-Chaikoff effect, with resultant goitre and hypothyroidism.

#73. e) All of the above
Iodine deficiency may predispose a patient to thyroid cancer, a goitre, toxic-multinodular goitre and cretinism in infants of pregnant mothers who are iodine depleted.

#74. d) 90-95%
Thyroid Incidentalomas are common findings at autopsies of elderly patients; a palpable nodule is present in 4-7% of the population (and a higher amount are impalpable). Nodules are more common in females (four times); however, this is countered by malignancy more likely in males. The vast majority are benign; only 5-10% are cancerous, however all must be investigated as it is difficult to know which of the 5-10% are cancerous.

#75. e) Serum TSH and T4
Thyroid function tests should be ordered after identification of a thyroid nodule; low TSH is suggestive of hyperthyroidism, for which a thyroid scintigraphy will be ordered (if 'hot', no further investigation is required as these are nearly always benign). Normal or increased TSH requires an ultrasound scan, which potential for a biopsy.

#76. b) Females
Thyroid nodules are four times more likely in females, and are furthermore associated with elderly patients, and in iodine-insufficient regions.

#77. e) Size above two centimetres
All of the listed options are 'red flags' apart from size; on its own, is not a 'red-flag' however a history of a rapid enlargement is concerning for malignancy.

#78. a) and c) (option e)
Sonographic features suggestive of a benign lesion include: Well-marginated, peripheral vascularity and hyperechoic appearance.

Sonographic features suggestive of malignancy include: Hypoechoic lesion, irregular margins, central blood flow, nodular height greater than width and macrocalcifications.

#79. c) Vitamin A
Hypothyroidism in the presence of iodine deficiency may be worsened by a co-existing deficiency of Vitamin A. Vitamin A modulates peripheral metabolism of thyroid hormones in addition to decreasing the production of TSH from the anterior pituitary gland. Therefore, Vitamin A deficiency leads to increased TSH stimulation and worsening of goitre from the absence of Vitamin A-mediated suppression of TSH-beta gene in the pituitary gland.

#80. d) Alcoholism
Rather strangely, moderate alcohol consumption is associated with a reduction in the risk of developing Graves' Disease. The underlying mechanism is unclear.

#81. b) Cowden Syndrome
Cowden Syndrome is an autosomal dominant disorder resulting in multiple hamartomas in addition to an increased risk for acquiring breast, thyroid and uterine cancer (amongst others).

#82. d) Thionamide treatment for five years
Longer-term treatment with thionamides (5-10 years) as opposed to the traditional 12-18 months of therapy are associated with a significant decrease in the likelihood of relapse. Males are more likely to relapse, however, in the post-partum period females are at an increased risk for relapse. Graves' Disease is more likely to relapse in the spring and summer months, as well as in patients with hay-fever (helper T cells subtype 2 worsen cytokine production).

#83. e) Upper-lid retraction
Upper-lid retraction is the earliest sign of Grave's Ophthalmopathy.

#84. b) Autoimmune Hypothyroidism
This vignette demonstrates Turner's Syndrome; patients with Turner's Syndrome are predisposed towards autoimmune hypothyroidism.

#85. c) Delayed relaxation of deep tendon reflexes
A peculiar physical sign of hypothyroidism is the slow and delayed relaxation phase of deep tendon reflexes

#86. b) 12 weeks
Foetal thyroid tissue begins to release thyroid hormones at 12 weeks, however, is still dependent upon maternal T4 until the mid-second trimester.

#87. b) Papillary Carcinoma
Orphan-Annie Nuclei are a characteristic histopathological sign suggestive of a papillary carcinoma; Orphan Annie Nuclei are large cells, with clear cytoplasm and dense nuclei.

#88. a) Follicular Carcinoma
A classic exam question: Papillary Carcinomas spread via the lymph route, whereas papillary carcinomas spread via the haematogenous route

#89. b) Medullary Thyroid Carcinoma
Semaglutide is known to increase the risk of developing medullary thyroid carcinoma; therefore, with a family history of multiple endocrine neoplasia this medication must be avoided.

#90. e) Anaplastic Carcinoma
This carcinoma of the thyroid demonstrates the poorest prognosis and is rapidly fatal. It is very uncommon, and most prevalent amongst elderly patients, as a rapidly enlarging anterior neck mass.

#91. c) Type 2 Diabetes Mellitus
Selenium Supplementation is recommended to treat mild graves' ophthalmopathy; it should be made clear to patients however, that there is an increase in the risk of acquiring type 2 diabetes mellitus.

#92. d) Teprotumumab
Teprotumumab is a monoclonal antibody functioning to inhibit the insulin-like growth factor 1 (IGF-1) receptor, approved for the treatment of moderate to severe Graves' Ophthalmopathy. Teprotumumab functions to displace IGF-1 from its receptor and promoting internalisation and degradation of both the receptor and receptor-antibody complexes. Side effects include hyperglycaemia,

fatigue, dysgeusia, headache, dry skin, hearing impairment, nausea, diarrhoea and muscle spasms.

#93. b) Inflammatory and Fibrotic
Thyroid Eye Disease typically follows two 'phases' – inflammatory and fibrotic. Medications are more effective during the active, inflammatory stage, whereas surgery is more likely required during the fibrotic stage.

#94. b) Thyroid Eye Disease
Rundle's Curve is used to graph the natural course of Thyroid Eye Disease.

#95. c) Widened Palpebral Fissure
Darlymple's Sign is best described as a widened palpebral fissure (commonest sign); this is one of many eponymous thyroid eye signs.

#96. b) Asians
It is important to note that Asian patients may demonstrate lower-lid (rather than the classic upper-lid) retraction.

#97. a) and c) (option e)
Recent evidence has suggested Thyroid Eye Disease should be the proper nomenclature (rather than Graves' Ophthalmopathy) as it can be present in both Hashimoto's Thyroiditis and Thyroid Cancer (albeit at a much lower prevalence).

#98. a) Intravenous Corticosteroids
Sight-threatening Graves' Ophthalmopathy requires hospital admission for intravenous corticosteroids and consideration for orbital decompression surgery.

#99. c) Euthyroid
This vignette describes post-partum thyroiditis, for which the majority of patients will recover without permanent thyroid disease.

#100. a) and d) (option e)
The vignette is suggestive of Riedel's (Fibrosing) Thyroiditis; this may occur on its own with thyroid involvement, or as part of wide-spread IgG4 disease. Retroperitoneal fibrosis, woody/hard thyroid tissue is a classic description.

#101. c) Aggravation of symptoms in the first half, followed by relaxation in the second half of pregnancy; these patients are at an increased risk of relapse post-partum

Females with Grave's Disease may experience aggravation of symptoms in the first half of pregnancy, followed by relaxation of symptoms; this is however, coupled with an increased risk for relapse in the post-partum period.

#102. a) Lingual Tissue

As the thyroid begins its descent from the foramen caecum of the tongue, this is the most common site for ectopic thyroid tissue (lingual thyroid); these patients must be assessed for functioning thyroid tissue prior to its removal, as this may be the only source and removal will render permanent hypothyroidism.

#103. b) Factitious Hyperthyroidism

Always consider factitious hyperthyroidism when a complete work-up reveals no likely cause. As with this vignette the patients are typically within the medical profession and may have easy means to obtain levothyroxine. Exogenous levothyroxine will lead to atrophy of the thyroid gland. Thyroid Scintigraphy will demonstrate diminished uptake – this can be difficult to distinguish from thyroiditis, however, factitious hyperthyroidism presents with decreased thyroglobulin in the serum.

#104. a) Alpha-subunit; Beta-subunit

All Glycoproteins (TSH, beta-HCG, FSH and LH) demonstrate a common alpha-subunit, however, it is the beta-subunit which demonstrates its specificity.

#105. b) McCune-Albright Syndrome

McCune Albright Syndrome is a genetic disorder (not-inherited), due to a mutation within the GNAS gene, coding for the stimulatory G-protein alpha-subunit. The resultant effect is constitutive activation of the receptor. The disorder is characterised by fibrous dysplasia of the bones, hyperfunctional endocrine organs and café-au-lait macules (hyperpigmented skin lesions). The endocrine manifestations may include precocious puberty, hyperthyroidism, hypothyroidism, gigantism and Cushing's syndrome (to name a few).

#106. d) Hashimoto's Thyroiditis
Elevated TSH (and TRH) is a stimulus for the release of prolactin; hypothyroidism must always be considered as a cause for hyperprolactinaemia.

#107. a) Pendred Syndrome
Pendred Syndrome is an autosomal recessive disorder characterised by a mutation in the PDS gene, coding for the protein Pendrin. Pendrin functions to transport iodide across the follicular cell's apical surface to the follicular lumen. Pendred Syndrome is characterised by sensorineural hearing loss (bilateral), goitre and mild hypothyroidism (or euthyroid).

#108. e) All of the above may be causal factors
All the options listed may be reasons for inadequate serum thyroxine despite adherence. Levothyroxine must be stored in a cool environment, and therefore at room temperatures may become unstable. Moreover, caution must be taken when switching to a generic version of a medication, as these demonstrate differing bioavailabilities. Many of the formulations may contain lactose, which may not be tolerated in a patient with severe lactose intolerance. Infrequently, anti-thyroxine autoantibodies may be present in a patient's serum; this can lead to either spuriously elevated or depressed levels of serum T4 depending upon the type of assay used.

#109. d) Testicular Germ Cell Tumour
This vignette describes a male patient with a prior history of cryptorchidism who is now presenting with systemic symptoms (such as weight loss). Moreover, he is demonstrating thyrotoxic symptomatology; in the presence of cryptorchidism, weight loss and thyrotoxic symptomatology in a male patient, one must consider a testicular tumour, which is hypersecreting beta-hCG.

#110. b) 15:1
The correct ratio of T4: T3 to prescribe when considering combination therapy is around 13-16:1. Commercially available combination medications are not appropriate as these demonstrate an inadequate ratio of 5:1, therefore the T4 and T3 are prescribed individually. Patients must be warned of the risks of precipitating an underlying arrhythmia and may lead to subclinical hyperthyroidism. There is limited long-term data regarding its safety, and it is furthermore not

appropriate in pregnant females. Liothyronine (T3) is very expensive, and hence clinicians must carefully identify the appropriate candidate, and discontinue if there is no subjective and/or objective benefit. Patients are to be made aware prior to commencing combination therapy that this is a 'therapeutic trial'.

#111. a) and d) (option e)
Administering growth hormone in a patient with growth hormone deficiency will lead to a decrease in free T4; therefore, if concurrently prescribed levothyroxine, the dosage of levothyroxine will likely need to be increased. Moreover, administering growth hormone in a euthyroid patient may occasionally 'unmask' central hypothyroidism. A deficiency of growth hormone may therefore 'mask' hypothyroidism, by keeping free T4 within the reference range. Similarly, in hypothyroidism, there is a reduction in secretion of both growth hormone and insulin-like growth factor 1, which may limit the usefulness of an insulin tolerance test (hypothyroidism must always be corrected beforehand). Although chronic, large doses of glucocorticoids may decrease serum TSH levels, this is not clinically significant and does not require an increase in dosage of levothyroxine. Oral oestrogen (such as the contraceptive pill) leads to an increase in thyroxine-binding globulin (TBG), to which an increased dose of levothyroxine is required to maintain free T4.

#112. c) Renal Failure
The dosage of levothyroxine can be decreased in lean patients (and increased in obese patients). Moreover, elderly patients demonstrated higher levels of TSH, for which does not necessarily necessitate an increased dosage. As elderly may harbour cardiovascular disease, a reduction in dosage may be more appropriate depending on the clinical picture. Although not studied in great detail, in female patients undergoing androgen administration for reasons such as breast cancer, there is a reversible effect with androgens, with a reduced dosage required for thyroid replacement.

#113. b) Soft-gel capsules
Apart from gelatin, allergies to the remaining fillers within levothyroxine tablets can be managed by administering soft-gel capsules, containing liquid T4.

<u>#114.</u> a) and d) (option e)
A gluten-free diet is the universal management of coeliac's disease; on its own this may result in improved absorption of levothyroxine. If absorption is still inadequate, soft-gel or liquid formulations are likely to overcome the resistance of absorption.

<u>#115.</u> a) and b) (option c)
The administration of levothyroxine is mandatory with a total thyroidectomy as there will be no residual thyroid tissue in the patient. Moreover, apart from the avoidance of hypothyroidism, it is hypothesised that decreased TSH prevents regrowth/recurrence of the thyroid carcinoma.

<u>#116.</u> a), b) and c) (option e)
Combination therapy may be attempted in patients with a diminished quality of life despite maximum levothyroxine adherence. Although there is not enough robust evidence to suggest screening for the DIO2 gene mutation in patients with hypothyroidism, those who are known to harbour a mutation and experience a diminished quality of life are candidates for combination therapy. In cases of myxoedema coma, many guidelines may recommend the administration of combination therapy (however, due to likely reduced gastrointestinal absorption, intravenous administration is suggested).

<u>#117.</u> c) Glucocorticoids inhibit the peripheral conversion of T4 to T3
Although glucocorticoids suppress TSH, this is unlikely in the acute setting and is typically insignificant. Glucocorticoids are prescribed in a thyroid storm as they reduce the conversion of T4 to T3 (similarly to propylthiouracil), in addition to enhancing stabilisation of the vascular system and likely reducing the autoimmune inflammatory response which led to the thyroid storm. In a manner similar to managing a myxoedema coma, glucocorticoids are also given in a thyroid storm as there may be an associated adrenal insufficiency.

<u>#118.</u> b) Cholestyramine
Cholestyramine, a bile-acid-sequestrant, may be prescribed in a thyroid storm, as it reduces the enterohepatic circulation of thyroid hormones.

<u>#119.</u> b) Riedel's Thyroiditis
Tamoxifen has proven effective in the management of Riedel's Thyroiditis, which is believed to occur separate to anti-oestrogenic

mechanisms. Tamoxifen promotes the release of Transforming-Growth-Factor Beta, which inhibits fibroblast proliferation.

#120. b), c) and d) (option e)
Turner's Syndrome (45, X0) and Down's Syndrome (Trisomy 21) are two well-established genetic disorders with an increased susceptibility towards acquiring autoimmune hypothyroidism. Although antithyroid antibodies are at a higher prevalence in Noonan's Syndrome, there is no increased risk of autoimmune hypothyroidism. Although iodine deficiency is a common cause of hypothyroidism, iodine excess can also cause hypothyroidism. In the healthy patient, this leads to the wolff-chaikoff effect, but after a few days this is no longer present as the normal thyroid tissue overcomes this blockade. In patients with pre-existing thyroid abnormalities, the iodine administration leads to hypothyroidism from which the gland cannot 'escape' from.

#121. d) Six Weeks
Levothyroxine demonstrates a half-life of around one week, therefore the steady state concentration (around six half-lives) is not present until around six weeks (for which the next measurement is recommended)

#122. f) All of the above are complications
Hypothyroidism is a well-known cause of persistently elevated LDL-cholesterol, which may be resistant to statin medications. Moreover, there is occasionally elevated serum creatine kinase; it is unknown why but likely due to abnormal myocyte metabolism and resultant dysfunction. Chronic hypothyroidism is associated with hyponatraemia, from increased levels of antidiuretic hormone. Microcytic anaemia may occur from prolonged menorrhagia. Macrocytic anaemia may occur either from the association of a second autoimmune condition such as Pernicious Anaemia, or as a result of uncertain mechanisms, likely due to disruption of the cell's lipid membrane.

#123. b) and c) (option e)
The right lobe is more vascular than the left, and therefore larger and more frequently enlarges in thyroid disorders. The pyramidal lobe is the distal remnant of the thyroglossal duct, which arises from the isthmus in most patients. It is present in a significant proportion of the general population (at least 33%) and is typically asymptomatic.

#124. b) Medullary Thyroid Carcinoma
Amyloid deposition within the tumour and surrounding tissues may occur with medullary thyroid carcinoma, as a result of calcitonin production.

#125. a) Tetany
Despite the function of calcitonin reducing the serum calcium levels, this is rarely of clinical significance. Calcitonin is typically asymptomatic, however, occasionally symptoms such as flushing, diarrhoea and pruritus may occur, and this may be indistinguishable from carcinoid syndrome. This is quite rare and may signify advanced (or metastatic) disease.

#126. d) Pyogenic Thyroiditis
An underlying pyriform sinus may lead to a fistula towards to thyroid, and in children this can present as pyogenic thyroiditis following an upper-respiratory tract infection. Management is directed towards the underlying infection (viral, fungal, bacterial) in addition to drainage of abscess (if developed) and/or surgical removal of the fistula.

#127. d) Excess thyroid hormones increase the production of sex-hormone binding globulin (SHBG)
Increase sex-hormone binding globulin leads to a relative deficiency of free testosterone (increased oestrogen to testosterone ratio), and therefore patients with hyperthyroidism may display gynaecomastia.
#128. d) Subclinical Hypothyroidism
The vignette is suggestive of subclinical hypothyroidism; do not be fooled into thinking subclinical = asymptomatic! As in this patient, there are occasionally symptoms, and if severe/interfering with life, require treatment with levothyroxine. As TSH levels are 'variable', however, it is recommended that a repeat TSH is performed in three months before diagnosing the condition.

#129. f) A 42-year-old female with a TSH of 7.2mU/L and recurrent of fatigue
In patients under 70 years of age, treatment is not typically initiated with a TSH under 10.0mU/L and observation with repeat testing is suggested; in the presence of the following however, treatment may be recommended:
> *o Severe hypothyroid symptomatology*
> *o Goitre*

o *Bipolar*
o *High risk of cerebrovascular disease*
o *Prior miscarriages/infertility*

Patients above the age of 70 should only be treated if the TSH is greater than 10.0mU/L; this is because the levels of TSH increase with age, and a TSH of 7.0mU/L in an 80-year-old patient (as an example) may in fact be normal, with administration of thyroxine causing unnecessary harm. If the TSH is above 10.0mU/L however, levothyroxine should be considered (typically if hypothyroid symptoms are present or there is a high vascular risk).

<u>#130.</u> c) and d) (option e)
The Suspensory Ligament of the Thyroid Gland, also referred to as Berry's Ligament, is a cluster of fascia (pre-tracheal fascia) which form to anchor the thyroid to posterior crico-tracheal structures.

<u>#131.</u> b) Slipped Capital Femoral Epiphysis
Slipped Capital Femoral Epiphysis is most common in young, obese male patients. Moreover, there may be an endocrinopathy, such as hypothyroidism. Slipped Capital Femoral Epiphysis is a misnomer, as the disorder occurs as a result of the metaphysis sliding anterior (however, imaging studies present what looks like posterior slippage of the epiphysis).

<u>#132.</u> e) Subclinical Hyperthyroidism
The vignette is descriptive for subclinical hyperthyroidism; do not be fooled into thinking subclinical hyperthyroidism must be asymptomatic! It is possible the refractory to therapy for atrial fibrillation is due to subclinical hyperthyroidism. A TSH below 0.01mU/L is very suggestive of a true thyroid axis anomaly such as subclinical hyperthyroidism rather than artefact or sick euthyroid syndrome. The level of TSH may be 'graded', whereby grade 1 incorporates 0.1-0.4mU/L, and grade 2 incorporating below 0.1mU/L. This patient therefore harbours grade 2 TSH; in addition to the increased age and cardiovascular risk factors, it is imperative to manage the underlying cause of the subclinical hyperthyroidism.

<u>#133.</u> a) Delphian Lymph Node
The Delphian Lymph Node is located above the thyroid isthmus and drains the upper poles of the thyroid gland and the larynx. Thyroid

carcinomas may metastasise to this node, which may be resected for a 'sentinel lymph node biopsy'._

#134. e) Tubercle of Zuckerkandl

The Tubercle of Zuckerkandl is present on the posterior surface of the thyroid gland, present in the majority of patients. This serves as a landmark for head and neck surgeons, as the recurrent laryngeal nerve passes medial to it.

#135. b) Brachiocephalic Trunk

The Thyroid Ima Artery most commonly arises from the brachiocephalic trunk.

#136. d) Acromegaly

One of the consequences of acromegaly is enlargement of the thyroid tissue, which leads to a goitre. The thyroid may be enlarged diffusely or multinodular. Thyroid function is most commonly normal, however, case reports have described subclinical hyperthyroidism, as well as central hypothyroidism (from tumour enlargement). There is a slightly increased prevalence of thyroid cancer amongst patients with acromegaly compared to the general population.

#137. e) Thyrotrophe Hyperplasia

Long-standing untreated hypothyroidism may lead to pituitary hyperplasia (of the thyrotrophe cells), which can be mistaken for a pituitary adenoma if a brain MRI is performed. This will, however, decrease in response to levothyroxine (unlike a pituitary adenoma).

#138. c) Hypothyroidism can lead to precocious puberty; when associated with ovarian cysts, this is known as van-Wyck-Grumbach Syndrome

Hypothyroidism is a cause of precocious puberty. This may be referred to as van-Wyck-Grumbach Syndrome, however this technically refers hypothyroidism, precocious puberty and ovarian cysts. The proposed pathophysiology includes cross-reactivity of the FSH receptor by elevated TSH.

#139. b) Cystinosis

Cystinosis is a lysosomal storage disorder resulting in lysosomal accumulation of cystine. This results in crystal formation throughout *most organs in the body, including the thyroid gland, leading to hypothyroidism.*

#140. c) Thalidomide
Rare case-reports have demonstrated patients treated with Thalidomide to develop hypothyroidism.

#141. b) Paraganglioma
Apart from medullary thyroid carcinoma, multiple endocrine neoplasia may also give rise to a thyroid paraganglioma.

#142. d) Multiple Myeloma
To the best of the author's knowledge, monoclonal proteins have been reported to interfere with thyroid hormone assays with false positive T3 levels (spurious t3 toxicosis) and falsely elevated TSH.

#143. c) Reassurance
This is a case vignette of palpation thyroiditis, whereby the excessive palpation (by the patient and physician) has led to the release of preformed hormones. Similar presentations may occur with trauma, known as traumatic thyroiditis. This is self-limiting and requires reassurance.

#144. d) Palpation Thyroiditis
See explanation for question #143.

#145. c) Ingestion of thyroid tissue
Hamburger thyrotoxicosis resulted from the strap muscles and thyroid tissue being consumed. Since then, more strict regulations have been put in place.

#146. d) TSH is not used in the first few month's post-initiation of medication
The TSH has been chronically suppressed and therefore will take up to six months to 'reawaken', therefore in the first few months the measurement is of little clinical value.

#147. b) and c) (option e)
This is a form of atrophic thyroiditis, which presents without a goitre. Moreover, the transient phase of thyrotoxicosis is not likely to be seen.

#148. d) Hyperthyroidism
Epoprostenol is an intravenous prostacyclin used in the treatment of pulmonary arterial hypertension. A known side-effect of this medication is hyperthyroidism, occurring in less than one percent of patients.

#149. d) Hyperthyroidism refers to hyperfunctioning thyroid tissue, whereas thyrotoxicosis refers to the clinical phenotype
It is important to note that many disorders, such as DeQuervain's Thyroiditis, are a cause of 'Thyrotoxicosis without Hyperthyroidism' as there is no underlying hyperfunctioning of the thyroid tissue.

#150. d) Uncontrolled hyperthyroidism in-utero
Cranial synostosis (Craniosynostosis) is the premature closure of the sutures of the skull. This is a known consequence of severe, uncontrolled hyperthyroidism in-utero.

#151. c) Follicular Carcinoma
Although extremely unlikely to lead to hyperthyroidism, metastatic follicular carcinoma has occasionally been depicted to lead to hyperfunctional thyroid tissue. More commonly however, cancers may lead to hyperthyroidism by compressing the thyroid tissue, known as Carcinomatous Thyroiditis.

#152. c) Cabbage, Cauliflower and Broccoli
These cruciferous vegetables contain metabolites that compete with iodine for thyroidal uptake, leading to the development of a goitre.

#153. c) Central Hypothyroidism
Bexarotene, used for Mycosis Fungoides, is known to increase the clearance of free T4 and decrease the release of TSH, leading to central hypothyroidism.

#154. a) Neurologic Cretinism
Neurologic cretinism is believed to be a result of early hypothyroidism in gestation, followed by euthyroid status post-natally.
Myxoedematous Cretinism, however, will present with hypothyroidism, and is likely a result of iodine deficiency and thyroid injury in the later part of pregnancy, continuing post-natally.

<u>#155.</u> b) Follicular
Fine needle aspiration cytology is unreliable for follicular carcinoma as only the cells are observed; naturally follicular carcinoma will demonstrate normal appearing follicular cells (moreover, difficult to differentiate follicular adenoma from carcinoma).

<u>#156.</u> e) Hyperthyroidism; Systolic Hypertension
This is a classic exam question; Hyperthyroidism increase the systolic blood pressure, whereas hypothyroidism increases the diastolic blood pressure.

<u>#157.</u> d) POEMS Syndrome
This condition is characterised by <u>P</u>olyneuropathy, <u>O</u>rganomegaly, <u>E</u>ndocrinopathy, <u>M</u>onoclonal Protein and <u>S</u>kin Changes. Hypothyroidism is a common endocrine association of POEMS Syndrome.

<u>#158.</u> b) Thionamide medications used in the management of hyperthyroidism may cause ANCA positive vasculitis
Thionamide medications may lead to a drug induced ANCA positive vasculitis. This is reversible upon discontinuation.

<u>#159.</u> e) Patients can breastfeed on either medication
The levels reaching the breast milk are of too little quantity to affect the neonatal thyroid tissue.

<u>#160.</u> c) Recovery from Sick Euthyroid Syndrome
Although Sick Euthyroid Syndrome may have a decreased TSH, the recovery phase may 'overshoot' the reference range and present with elevated serum TSH. It is much more common that an ill patient in the hospital has elevated TSH as a result of 'recovery' from sick euthyroid syndrome than of true hypothyroidism.

Pituitary Gland & Hypothalamus

#1. 'Pituitary' is derived from the latin word 'pituitarius', referring to the release of phlegm. This organ was previously believed to release phlegm which drained through the nose. Nowadays, this is known to be incorrect, and the pituitary gland is divided into an anterior portion, and a posterior portion. All of the following hormones are released from the anterior pituitary gland except for:

      a) Prolactin
      b) Growth Hormone
      c) Thyrotrophin
      d) Oxytocin
      e) Adrenocorticotrophic Hormone

#2. The posterior pituitary gland, unlike its anterior counterpart, does not receive a concentrated influx of releasing hormones from the hypothalamus. Instead, the posterior pituitary gland is in direct neuroconnection with the hypothalamic nuclei, leading to the release of its respective hormones. Which of the following options correctly pairs the posterior pituitary hormones and their respective hypothalamic nuclei?

      a) Median Eminence (Vasopressin); Periventricular Nuclei (Prolactin)
      b) Periventricular Nuclei (Prolactin); Supraventricular Nuclei (Vasopressin)
      c) Paraventricular Nuclei (Vasopressin); Supraoptic Nuclei (Oxytocin)
      d) Infraoptic Nuclei (Prolactin); Periventricular Nuclei (Vasopressin)
      e) Supraoptic Nuclei (Vasopressin); Paraventricular Nuclei (Oxytocin)

#3. Which of the following anatomical structures is located laterally to the pituitary gland?

      a) Optic Chiasm
      b) Sphenoid Sinus
      c) Sella Turcica
      d) Cavernous Sinus
      e) Pterygoid Sinus

#4. The anterior pituitary gland, also known as the adenohypophysis, has a direct continuation of blood supply (hypophyseal portal circulation) from the hypothalamus. The portal circulation, derived from the superior hypophyseal artery, is a branch of which of the following arteries?

       a) External Carotid Artery
       b) Subclavian Artery
       c) Vertebral Artery
       d) Internal Carotid Artery
       e) Maxillary Artery

#5. The posterior pituitary gland, alternatively referred to as the neurohypophysis, receives its blood supply from the inferior hypophyseal artery. Which of the following options correctly identifies the origins of this artery?

       a) Meningohypophyseal trunk
       b) Internal thoracic artery
       c) External Carotid Artery
       d) Vertebral Artery
       e) None of the above

#6. Despite the differences in arterial supply to the anterior and posterior pituitary glands, there is a common venous drainage system. The venous drainage flows into the cavernous sinus, followed by the petrosal sinuses and eventually reaching the jugular bulb. Inferior Petrosal Sinus sampling (IPSS) is most frequently used as an intervention to determine which of the following?

       a) Cushing's Disease
       b) Thyrotrophinoma
       c) Acromegaly
       d) Syndrome of Inappropriate Antidiuretic Hormone (SIADH)
       e) Prolactinoma

#7. A 32-year-old Multigravida at 39 weeks delivers a healthy infant boy. The vaginal delivery is complicated by uterine atony and a resultant post-partum haemorrhage protocol is initiated. She is managed with oxytocin, haemabate and the insertion of a urinary catheter and subsequently begins to recover. Over the following three days however, she is unable to breast-feed; she had no difficulty with her prior children. Which of the following is the most likely diagnosis?

a) Lymphocytic Hypophysitis
b) Sheehan's Syndrome
c) Pituitary Apoplexy
d) Empty Sella syndrome

#8. With reference to question #7, which of the following options correctly suggests the effects upon the posterior pituitary gland?
a) The posterior pituitary gland is equally affected; however, symptoms are more subtle and not routinely tested for
b) The posterior pituitary gland is unaffected as it functions under a low-pressure system
c) The posterior pituitary gland is more often affected than the anterior pituitary gland
d) The posterior pituitary gland is unaffected as it functions under a high-pressure system
e) None of the above are correct

#9. Although adjacent, the embryological origins of both the adenohypophysis and neurohypophysis are different. Around week four of gestation, Rathke's Pouch begins to develop from the oral ectoderm, eventually separating at the end of the second month of gestation and reaching the neural cavity. A remnant of Rathke's Pouch may occasionally transform into a neoplasm with a characteristic calcification upon imaging. This mass furthermore is distinct from other childhood cranial neoplasms, as it is located supra-tentorially, whilst most childhood intracranial neoplasms are infra-tentorial. Which of the following options correctly identifies this mass?
a) Eosinophilic Granuloma
b) Hand-Schüller-Christian Disease
c) Craniopharyngioma
d) Rathke cleft cyst
e) Arachnoid cyst

#10. Around which week of gestation is there evidence of 'primitive' hormonal production from the anterior pituitary gland.
a) Seven Weeks
b) Twelve Weeks
c) Seventeen Weeks
d) 32 Weeks
e) Post-partum

<u>#11.</u> The adenohypophysis comprises what percentage of the pituitary gland?

- a) 10%
- b) 20%
- c) 40%
- d) 50%
- e) 80%

<u>#12.</u> The anterior wall of the adenohypophysis is divided into the pars distalis, with the upward growth of the anterior wall forming the pars tuberalis, surrounding the infundibulum. The posterior wall forms which of the following portions of the anterior pituitary gland?

- a) Pars Inferioris
- b) Pars Nervosa
- c) Pars Intermedia
- d) Pars Nodosa
- e) There is no posterior wall

<u>#13.</u> With reference to question #12, which of the following hormones is believed to be released from this portion of the anterior pituitary gland (and is hypertrophied in pregnancy)?

- a) Prolactin
- b) Growth Hormone
- c) Melanocyte-Stimulating Hormone
- d) Thyroid-Stimulating Hormone
- e) None of the above

<u>#14.</u> With the development of the adenohypophysis, there is simultaneous development of the neurohypophysis. Unlike the adenohypophysis, the neurohypophysis grows **downward**, from the diencephalon (posterior area of the forebrain) and attaches to the anterior pituitary gland at around week five. The Infundibulum (as a result of descent) further gives rise to the pituitary stalk and which of the following portions of the posterior pituitary gland?

- a) Pars Inferioris
- b) Pars Nervosa
- c) Pars Intermedia
- d) Pars Nodosa
- e) Pars Tuberalis

#15. Which of the following cell types in the anterior pituitary gland are the most numerous (50% of cells), and is the first to be lost in the hypopituitarism sequence?

    a) Thyrotrophes
    b) Lactotrophes
    c) Gonadotrophes
    d) Somatotrophes
    e) Corticotrophes

#16. Which of the following is the least numerous cell type within the anterior pituitary gland?

    a) Thyrotrophes
    b) Lactotrophes
    c) Gonadotrophes
    d) Somatotrophes
    e) Corticotrophes

#17. With a macroadenoma leading to 'mass-effect' and progressive hypopituitarism, which of the following is the last hormone the be affected in the hypopituitarism sequence?

    a) Thyrotrophes
    b) Lactotrophes
    c) Gonadotrophes
    d) Somatotrophes
    e) Corticotrophes

#18. Histochemical staining of pituitary cells of the anterior pituitary gland delineates three predominant categories: Acidophils, Basophils and Chromophobes. Which of the following options correctly pairs the cell types and their respective function?

    a) Acidophil: Release Glycopeptides; Basophils: Release Polypeptides; Chromophobes: Release either Glycopeptides or Polypeptides
    b) Acidophil: Release Polypeptides; Basophils: Release Glycopeptides; Chromophobes: Release either Glycopeptides or Polypeptides
    c) Acidophil: Release Glycopeptides; Basophils: Release Polypeptides; Chromophobes: Do not release any hormone

d) Acidophil: Release Polypeptides; Basophils: Release Glycopeptides; Chromophobes: Do not release any hormone

#19. Acidophils constitute around 40% of cells within the anterior pituitary, with Basophils constituting around 10%. Which of the following options correctly identifies an acidophilic cell-type paired with a basophilic cell-type?

a) Somatotrophes; Lactotrophes
b) Lactotrophes; Somatotrophes
c) Thyrotrophes; Lactotrophes
d) Gonadotrophes; Somatotrophes
e) Somatotrophes; Thyrotrophes

#20. The release of prolactin is under the inhibitory control of which chemical messengers (tuberoinfundibular pathway of the hypothalamus)?

a) Somatostatin
b) Prolactin-Inhibiting Hormone
c) Dopamine
d) a) and c)
e) b) and c)

#21. All of the following hormones are glycoproteins except for which of the following?

a) Gonadotrophes
b) Thyrotrophes
c) Lactotrophes
d) Corticotrophes

#22. Each glycoprotein has an alpha and beta subunit. Which of the following options correctly denotes the functions of these subunits?

a) Alpha subunit determines specificity; Beta-subunit is the common ancestral subunit
b) Alpha subunit is the common ancestral subunit and determines specificity; Beta-subunit functions for plasma stabilisation
c) Alpha subunit is the common ancestral subunit; Beta-subunit functions for plasma stabilisation
d) Alpha subunit is the common ancestral subunit; Beta-subunit functions to determine specificity

e) Alpha-subunit functions for plasma stability;
Beta-subunit is the common ancestral subunit

#23. Elevated levels of alpha-subunit in the serum are used to diagnose which of the following pituitary disorders?
a) Pituitary Resistance to Thyroid Hormones
b) Pituitary Resistance to TRH
c) Thyrotrophinoma
d) Pituitary Apoplexy
e) Heterophile Antibody Interference

#24. Adrenocorticotrophic Hormone is a breakdown product of Pro-opiomelanocortin (POMC) along with which of the following hormones?
a) Alpha-Melanocyte-Stimulating Hormone
b) Beta-Endorphin
c) Gamma-Melanocyte-Stimulating Hormone
d) a) and b)
e) a), b) and c)

#25. Gonadotrophes, known to release luteinizing hormone (LH) and follicle stimulating hormone (FSH) may undergo hypertrophy in which of the following clinical conditions?
a) Hyperprolactinaemia
b) Secondary Gonadal Failure
c) Primary Gonadal Failure
d) All of the above

#26. Both Craniopharyngiomas and pituitary adenomas may give rise to Bitemporal Hemianopia and may occasionally lead to confusion in differentiating the two disorders. There is a subtle difference in the **initial** visual change, however this is often unnoticed by the patient until they have developed complete bitemporal hemianopia. Which of the following correctly suggests the initial visual presentations of the disorders?
a) A craniopharyngioma may initially present with unilateral homonymous hemianopia
b) A pituitary adenoma may initially present with inferior bitemporal hemianopia
c) A craniopharyngioma may initially present with inferior bitemporal hemianopia

    d) A pituitary adenoma may initially present with
       superior bitemporal hemianopia
    e) c) and d)
    f) a) and b)

#27. The commonest pituitary tumour overall is which of the
following?

    a) Prolactinoma
    b) Somatomammotrophinoma
    c) Gonadotrophinoma
    d) Non-functioning adenoma
    e) Metastasis

#28. The most common functioning pituitary adenoma is which of the
following?

    a) Corticotrophinoma
    b) Thyrotrophinoma
    c) Prolactinoma
    d) Somatotrophinoma
    e) Gonadotrophinoma

#29. All of the following anterior pituitary hormones are stimulated by
a hypothalamic-releasing factor except for which of the following:

    a) TSH
    b) ACTH
    c) FSH and LH
    d) Prolactin
    e) GH

#30. Which of the following options correctly identifies the gland
responsible for releasing melatonin?

    a) Anterior Pituitary Gland
    b) Posterior Pituitary Gland
    c) Pineal Gland
    d) Suprachiasmatic Nucleus of the Hypothalamus
    e) c) and d)

#31. The involvement of the gland listed in question #30 may lead to a
constellation of symptoms including loss of vertical up-gaze,
nystagmus (convergence retraction), diplopia and hyporeflexia of the
pupils. What is the medical condition described?

a) Phencyclidine Overdose
b) Progressive Supranuclear Palsy
c) Parinaud's Syndrome
d) Multiple Sclerosis
e) Argyll-Robertson Pupil

#32. A 75-year-old gentleman presents to his endocrine clinic with a six-week history of headaches and tiredness. He past medical history is unremarkable, and he does not take any medication. He is a retired solicitor and lives at home with his wife and eldest daughter. Upon further questioning, he embarrassingly admits to a decreased level of libido and erectile dysfunction. The physician performs a visual-field assessment, which is normal. An Anterior Pituitary Hormone Panel is performed, of which the results are demonstrated below:

Prolactin	815mU/L (Ref:45-400mU/L)
Free T4	15pmol/L (Ref: 12-22pmol/L)
TSH	2.2mU/L (Ref: 0.27-4.2mU/L)
FSH	7U/L (Ref: 1.6-11U/L)
LH	4U/L (Ref: 1.5-8U/L)
IGF-1	3nmol/L (Ref: 7-25nmol/L)
Testosterone	5nmol/L (Ref: 8-29nmol/L)
8AM Cortisol	380nmol/L (140-630nmol/L)
MRI Pituitary (Contrast)	Sellar mass (2cmx2cm) impinging optic chiasm

Which of the following is the most likely diagnosis?
a) Pituitary Macroadenoma
b) Pituitary Infarction
c) Pituitary Microadenoma
d) Non-functioning adenoma

#33. Which of the following is the correct explanation for the low testosterone in the above vignette?
a) Tumour expansion compressing gonadotrophes
b) Hyperprolactinaemia inhibition of gonadotrophes
c) The low testosterone is expected at his age (andropause)
d) a) and b)

#34. With reference to question #32, one week later the physician requests a repeat sample of prolactin using a different assay. The laboratory technician calls the physician and explains that the latest prolactin measurement is 6,000 mU/L. Which of the following is the most likely diagnosis assuming this is the correct prolactin level?

    a)   Pituitary Macroadenoma
    b)   Pituitary Infarction
    c)   Pituitary Microadenoma
    d)   Macroprolactin
    e)   Non-functioning adenoma

#35. Despite its name, histologically, most non-functional adenomas can be traced to which of the following anterior pituitary cell types?

    a)   Thyrotrophes
    b)   Gonadotrophes
    c)   Corticotrophes
    d)   Somatotrophes
    e)   Lactotrophes

#36. Approximately what percentage of the population will harbour a pituitary incidentaloma?

    a)   1%
    b)   10%
    c)   50%
    d)   50%
    e)   90%

#37. During a lecture for first-year medical students, a learned professor discusses the various types of pituitary adenomas. A student in the front-row asks at what diameter is an adenoma considered 'micro' or 'macro'?

    a)   10cm
    b)   1cm
    c)   5cm
    d)   5mm
    e)   Distinction is based on symptomatology, not a
         specific size

#38. All of the following pituitary adenomas require surgery as first-line, except for which of the following (for which medication is used first-line)?

    a)   Thyrotrophinoma
    b)   Acromegaly
    c)   Cushing's Disease

d) Prolactinoma
e) Non-functional adenoma

#39. Which of the following options correctly identifies the sequential loss of pituitary hormones in hypopituitarism?
a) GH > LH & FSH > TSH> ACTH
b) GH > TSH > LH & FSH > ACTH
c) TSH > GH > LH & FSH > ACTH
d) LH & FSH > GH > TSH > ACTH
e) GH > LH & FSH > ACTH > TSH

#40. In the presence of a non-functional macroadenoma, all of the following are absolute indications for surgery except for:
a) Symptomatic Hypopituitarism
b) Visual Field Defects
c) Mass Compressing/Approximating Optic Chiasm
d) Apoplexy
e) Headache

#41. Which of the following immunohistochemistry markers can be used to determine the progression, recurrence and malignancy risk of a pituitary adenoma?
a) Ki-23
b) Ki-63
c) Ki-67
d) Chromogranin

#42. A 34-year-old female presents to her family physician with a four-month history of intractable headaches. Her only past medical history is depression, for which she has been prescribed Sertraline for the past six months and is compliant with her prescription. She has explained to the physician that she has noted a loss of libido in the past few weeks. The physician is unfamiliar with the recommended guidelines, and commences an anterior pituitary hormone panel, demonstrated below.

Prolactin	400mU/L (Ref:60-620mU/L)
Free T4	15pmol/L (Ref: 12-22pmol/L)
TSH	2.2mU/L (Ref: 0.27-4.2mU/L)
FSH	6U/L (Ref: 3-11U/L)
LH	4U/L (Ref: 2-8U/L)
IGF-1	20nmol/L (Ref: 13-33nmol/L)
8AM Cortisol	500nmol/L (140-630nmol/L)

The physician subsequently requests an MRI of the pituitary with contrast. The report suggests a 6mm pituitary lesion with no shift of the pituitary stalk and away from the optic chiasm. Which of the following is the most likely diagnosis?

        a) Microprolactinoma
        b) Incidentaloma
        c) Macroprolactinoma
        d) Non-functional macroadenoma

#43. The patient in question #42 requests surgical removal of her mass, as the headaches have not improved with paracetamol. Which of the following is the correct response?

        a) The headache is unrelated to the tumour
        b) The headache is directly caused by the tumour
        c) Removal of the tumour will improve the headache
        d) Tumour size does not correlate with headache; there is no guarantee that surgery will improve the headache

#44. Which of the following differentiates Chiari-Frommel Syndrome from Ahumada-del Castillo syndrome?

        a) Chiari-Frommel occurs in the presence of a pituitary adenoma; Ahumada-del Castillo presents females who have recently given birth
        b) Chiari-Frommel occurs in females who have recently given birth; Ahumada-del Castillo presents in the presence of a pituitary adenoma
        c) Chiari-Frommel occurs in females who have recently given birth; Ahumada-del Castillo presents without recent delivery
        d) Chiari-Frommel presents without recent delivery; Ahumada-del Castillo presents in females who have recently given birth

#45. Which of the following options correctly identifies the following descriptive vignette: *An infrequent type of headache, which can occur from a posterior cranial fossa abnormality or pituitary adenoma. Symptoms include unilateral stabbing pain/burning around the eye, with autonomic symptoms (such as lacrimation, conjunctival injection,*

    a) SUNCT Headache (Short-lasting, unilateral neuralgiform headache attacks with conjunctival injection and tearing)
    b) SUNA (Short-lasting, unilateral neuralgiform headache attacks with cranial autonomic symptoms)
    c) Cluster headaches
    d) Paroxysmal Hemicrania
    e) Ice-Pick Headache

#46. What percentage of micro-incidentalomas will enlarge to become macro-incidentalomas?

    a) 10%
    b) 30%
    c) 50%
    d) 70%
    e) Virtually all will enlarge

#47. Which of the following scoring systems is used to grade the invasion of the cavernous sinus by a pituitary adenoma?

    a) Knosp Classification System
    b) SIPAP
    c) Hardy Classification
    d) None of the above

#48. A 66-year-old gentleman with acromegaly is scheduled for a transsphenoidal resection. His past medical history is significant for type 2 diabetes mellitus, controlled with pioglitazone and metformin. After removal of the tumour, the patient is noted to demonstrate an improvement in his glycaemic status, however, frequent hypoglycaemic episodes begin to occur. Which of the following is the terminology of this phenomenon?

    a) Geraldo's Phenomenon
    b) Houssay's Phenomenon
    c) Homer's Phenomenon
    d) Diabetes Paradox

#49. A 26-year-old female is referred to the Endocrinology Department at her local hospital after her general practitioner identified an elevated prolactin measurement of 1,100U/L. She does not take any medications and does not suffer from any conditions. She denies galactorrhoea, changes in menstrual cycle or headache. On examination she has a normal visual field assessment. The endocrinologist decides to perform a full anterior pituitary hormone panel, in addition to an MRI, demonstrated below.

Prolactin	1,100mU/L (Ref:60-620mU/L)
Free T4	19pmol/L (Ref: 12-22pmol/L)
TSH	3.8mU/L (Ref: 0.27-4.2mU/L)
FSH	16U/L (Ref: 3-11U/L)
LH	5U/L (Ref: 2-8U/L)
IGF-1	30nmol/L (Ref: 16-40nmol/L)
8AM Cortisol	600nmol/L (140-630nmol/L)
MRI Pituitary Contrast:	No abnormalities identified

Which of the following is the most likely diagnosis?
- a) Non-functioning microadenoma
- b) Microprolactinoma
- c) Macroprolactin
- d) Ectopic Secretion of Prolactin
- e) None of the above

#50. Which of the following structures listed does **not** pass through the cavernous sinus?
- a) Oculomotor Nerve
- b) Ophthalmic Division of the Trigeminal Nerve
- c) Internal Carotid Artery
- d) Abducens Nerve
- e) Mandibular Division of the Trigeminal Nerve
- f) Internal Carotid Artery
- g) Trochlear Nerve

#51. Knowledge of the surrounding structures of the sella turcica is of utmost importance. Which of the following structures is likely compressed in an expanding pituitary macroadenoma, when patients present with anosmia and an altered personality?
- a) Cribriform Plate
- b) Amygdala
- c) Frontal Lobe
- d) Parietal Lobe
- e) Nasal Cavity

#52. In around one-quarter of cases, Growth-Hormone secreting adenomas will additionally secrete which of the following?

a)   Prolactin
b)   TSH
c)   ACTH
d)   hCG
e)   FSH or LH

#53. The posterior pituitary gland is relatively unharmed from pituitary adenomas; typically, cranial diabetes insipidus will not manifest as vasopressin can be released from the hypothalamus. In which of the following clinical scenarios would cranial diabetes insipidus be present?

a)   Pituitary Metastases
b)   Traumatic Brain Injury
c)   Langerhan Cell Histiocytosis
d)   Stalk Compression
e)   Craniopharyngioma
f)   All of the above

#54. A 62-year-old male with unremitting headaches is demonstrated to be harbouring a non-functioning macroadenoma. Due to his religious beliefs, he refuses surgery or medication, believing the tumour will cure itself. The physician explains six-monthly MRI scans will be requested to monitor the growth. Whereas only around 10% of microadenomas will enlarge over the following decade, what is the likelihood for enlargement of macroadenomas over the next decade?

a)   0-10%
b)   30%-50%
c)   70-90%
d)   Virtually 100%

#55. Although classically taught in medical school that there are only three types of multiple endocrine neoplasia (types 1, 2A and 2B), many authors conclude there is additionally multiple endocrine neoplasia type 4. Which of the following options below correctly depicts the components of this syndrome?

a)   Parathyroid Adenoma; Pituitary Adenoma; Papillary Carcinoma
b)   Parathyroid Adenoma, Insulinoma, Medullary Thyroid Carcinoma

c) Parathyroid Adenoma, Pituitary Adenoma, Testicular Carcinoma
d) Multiple Endocrine Neoplasia Type 4 does not exist

#56. Which of the listed options correctly identifies the familial syndrome described: *Autosomal Recessive disorder, characterised by short stature, micropenis, hypoglycaemia and craniofacial abnormalities. Levels of IGF-1 are depleted in these patients; however, GH levels are elevated. Research suggests that despite these patients being obese, they are at a reduced risk for developing type 2 diabetes mellitus and cancer. The condition was originally described amongst patients of semitic ancestry, notably Sephardic Jews in Israel in 1966.*

a) Achondroplasia
b) Rhizomelic Chondrodysplasia Punctata
c) Pseudoachondroplasia
d) Leprechaunism
e) Laron-Type Dwarfism

#57. Which of the following options correctly identifies the effects both smoking and alcohol elicit upon the plasma osmolality?

a) Alcohol increases the release of vasopressin from the posterior pituitary gland; smoking inhibits the release of vasopressin
b) Both Alcohol and Smoking inhibit the release of vasopressin from the posterior pituitary gland
c) Both Alcohol and Smoking increase the release of vasopressin from the posterior pituitary gland
d) Alcohol inhibits the release of vasopressin from the posterior pituitary gland; Smoking increases the release of vasopressin from the posterior pituitary gland

#58. Mutations in the V2 Vasopressin receptor have been linked to familial forms of nephrogenic diabetes insipidus. The V2 receptor functions through the G-protein (stimulatory) pathway to increase the insertion of aquaporin 2, for which water can be reabsorbed. Which of the following options correctly identifies a substance released from Weibel-Palade bodies of the endothelium through the V2 receptor?

a) Factor V
b) Factor IX

c) von-Willebrand Factor
d) Tissue Factor III
e) Thrombin

#59. The V1 vasopressin receptor demonstrates which of the following effects?
a) Smooth muscle dilatation (Gi)
b) Aquaporin-4 Insertion (Gq)
c) Aquaporin-2 degradation (Gq)
d) Smooth muscle contraction (Gq)
e) None of the above

#60. Vasopressin may increase the release of which of the following anterior pituitary hormones?
a) TSH
b) ACTH
c) LH or FSH
d) Prolactin
e) GH

#61. A visiting medical student asks the consultant the following: *"if a single serum Growth Hormone level returns normal, can acromegaly be ruled out?"* Which of the following is the correct response?
a) Only in children
b) Only in adults
c) No; Acromegaly can still be present due to the pulsatile release of growth hormone from the pituitary gland.
d) If three consecutive levels return normal, acromegaly can be ruled out

#62. The same medical student in question #61 then proceeds to ask the following: *"Does this mean that a single TSH level should not be used to measure thyroid dysfunction?"* Which of the following is the correct response?
a) TSH should only be used to monitor secondary hypothyroidism, it has no value in primary hypothyroidism
b) TSH is only of value in hypothyroidism, not hyperthyroidism

144

c) Due to the short half-life of TSH and high amplitude of pulses, one level is not demonstrative of the underlying pathology
d) Due to the long-half-life of TSH and the low amplitude of pulses, one measurement is satisfactory to assess the underlying thyroid pathology

#63. Which of the following options correctly suggests the association between cushing's disease and the gonadotrophe cells?

a) Mass effect from pituitary adenoma, compressing gonadotrophe cells
b) Corticosteroids inhibit the release of gonadotrophins
c) FSH and LH receptors in the adrenal cortex promote the release of cortisol
d) All of the above may occur

#64. Which of the following hormones may be measured to differentiate a true seizure from a pseudoseizure?

a) Oxytocin
b) Prolactin
c) Cortisol
d) TSH
e) Growth Hormone

#65. Ghrelin, the 'hunger' hormone, is a stimulus for the release of which of the following anterior pituitary hormones?

a) Growth Hormone
b) Prolactin
c) TSH
d) ACTH
e) a) and d)

#66. A 32-year-old female with a six-month history of amenorrhoea presents to her general practitioner. On further history taking, the patient reveals recurrent headaches, and malaise. She has been diagnosed with depression one-year-ago after her long-term boyfriend ended their relationship, however, does not take any medication. She was prescribed combined oral contraceptive pills over the past five years, however, upon discontinuing one year-ago, her periods have not returned. She denies any nipple discharge, however, admits to a four-kilogram weight gain over the past year.

On examination, visual fields are unremarkable, and breast examination does not elicit discharge. There is no hirsutism or cushingoid appearance. The physician requests the following investigations:

Prolactin	2,100mU/L (Ref:60-620mU/L)
Free T4	21pmol/L (Ref: 12-22pmol/L)
TSH	4mU/L (Ref: 0.27-4.2mU/L)
FSH	9U/L (Ref: 3-11U/L)
LH	6U/L (Ref: 2-8U/L)
IGF-1	20nmol/L (Ref: 14-33nmol/L)
Oestradiol	115pmol/L (135-800nmol/L)
MRI Pituitary Non-Contrast:	No lesion identified; normal pituitary stalk

What is the most likely diagnosis?
  a) Macroprolactin
  b) Non-functioning microadenoma
  c) Hypothyroidism
  d) Medication-induced
  e) Microprolactinoma
  f) 'Idiopathic Hyperprolactinaemia' (Hyperprolactinaemia of Uncertain Aetiology)
  g) e) and f)

#67. All of the following are causes of raised prolactin except for:
  a) Renal Failure
  b) Liver Failure
  c) Pregnancy
  d) Polycystic Ovarian Syndrome
  e) Excessive Venipuncture Stress
  f) Ectopic Prolactin Secretion (e.g. RCC, CRC, Uterine Tumour)
  g) All of the above will increase prolactin levels

#68. Which of the following medications is not used in the management of a prolactinoma?
  a) Combined Oral Contraceptive Pill
  b) Bromocriptine
  c) Cabergoline
  d) Pasireotide

#69. Which of the following dopamine agonists is considered teratogenic and must not be taken during pregnancy (or in women seeking fertility)?

- a) Bromocriptine
- b) Cabergoline
- c) Quinagolide

#70. Around 15% of patients initially started on bromocriptine (the most researched dopamine agonist) will be resistant to the medication. Which of the following is true of this phenomenon?

- a) The patients are likely to be resistant to all dopamine agonists
- b) The patients likely harbour a non-functional adenoma, not a prolactinoma
- c) The patients require surgery
- d) The patients are likely to respond to cabergoline

#71. Which of the following dopamine agonists has the least side effects associated with it?

- a) Bromocriptine
- b) Cabergoline
- c) Quinagolide

#72. Although Cabergoline demonstrates a higher efficacy in normalising serum prolactin levels as well as decreasing the tumour size (compared to Bromocriptine), which of the following effects is a potential concern of Cabergoline?

- a) Myocardial Infarction
- b) Drug-Induced Parkinsonism
- c) Valvular Fibrosis
- d) Teratogenic
- e) All of the above

#73. With reference to question #72, through which receptor does this adverse effect occur?

- a) $5\text{-}HT_1$
- b) $5\text{-}HT_{2A}$
- c) $5\text{-}HT_{2B}$
- d) D_2
- e) D_4

<u>#74.</u> Around 20% of patients (males > females) will be resistant to dopamine agonists when treating a prolactinoma. It is believed the adenoma down-regulates the levels of available D_2 receptors, with macroadenomas more likely to be resistant over microadenomas. Resistance can only be 'labelled' when all available dopamine agonists have been trialled and are unsuccessful. Which of the following options correctly defines 'Dopamine Agonist Resistance'?

    a)   Failure to normalise prolactin
    b)   Failure to decrease adenoma size to below 50%
    c)   Failure to restore fertility in patients receiving standard dose
    d)   a) and b)
    e)   a), b) and c)

<u>#75.</u> A 35-year-old female, managed with bromocriptine for six-months, would like to know if she can stop taking her medication in the near future, as she would prefer to be off her medication in the long-term. Which of the following is the correct response?

    a)   Dopamine agonists cannot be taken for more than five years
    b)   Upon discontinuation of a dopamine agonist, serum prolactin is unlikely to increase
    c)   Upon discontinuation of a dopamine agonist, the adenoma is unlikely to increase
    d)   Dopamine agonists may be discontinued after two years if normoprolactinaemia is present in addition to the absence of a visible tumour on an MRI

<u>#76.</u> Which of the following is the correct advice to give a patient on bromocriptine for a microprolactinoma, in whom a pregnancy test returns positive?

    a)   Medication to be discontinued, as less than 5% of microadenomas will enlarge during pregnancy (risk of enlargement due to both oestrogen stimulation and withdrawal of medication). Patients to be followed-up in each trimester
    b)   Medication can be continued, as up to 30% of microprolactinomas may enlarge; visual fields

and MRI (non-contrast) performed in each
trimester
c)   Medication should be discontinued as is
teratogenic; prolactin should be measured
throughout pregnancy as this will correlate with
tumour size

<u>#77.</u> What is the correct advice to give to a primigravida mother with an asymptomatic microadenoma who would like to commence breastfeeding?

a)   Dopamine Agonists may be used during breast-feeding; the amount reaching the breast milk is minimal
b)   Breast-feeding is discouraged, as the adenoma may increase in growth
c)   Dopamine Agonists are discouraged as they inhibit lactation
d)   Dopamine agonists should be continued if they were required ruing pregnancy, and/or patient has visual filed impairment
e)   c) and d)

<u>#78.</u> The chance of remission of a microadenoma after pregnancy is roughly what percentage?

a)   0%-20%
b)   20-40%
c)   40-60%
d)   60-80%
e)   Around 100%

<u>#79.</u> A 63-year-old retired accountant presents to his family physician with the concern of 'visual problems'. He has recently noted that he keeps bumping into people whilst shopping, as well as nearly hitting parked cards on the street which he does not see. Further questioning suggests that he has a loss of libido and episodic headaches. He is not too concerned regarding his loss of libido, as him and his wife infrequently have intercourse. On physical examination, a visual field defect is identified as bitemporal hemianopia; an MRI with contrast confirms a pituitary mass impinging upon the optic chiasm. His serum prolactin is measured and returns elevated at 5,000mU/L. Which of the following is the first-line treatment?

a) Temozolomide
b) Dopamine Agonist
c) Transsphenoidal Surgery
d) Radiotherapy

#80. With reference to question #79, whilst undergoing treatment, he experiences a sudden, severe headache and loses consciousness. Upon reawakening, he is noted to have double vision, neck stiffness and clear fluid dripping from his nostrils. Which of the following options correctly pairs the likely diagnosis and management?

a) Epidural Haematoma; Neurosurgical Evacuation
b) Subarachnoid Haemorrhage; Calcium Channel Blockers
c) Sheehan's Syndrome; Blood Transfusion
d) Empty Sella syndrome; Neurosurgical Evacuation
e) Pituitary Apoplexy; Neurosurgical Evacuation

#81. A 69-year-old retired army general presents to his general practitioner with an unremitting headache and loss of libido. The gentleman is found to have bitemporal hemianopia on examination. Concerned that this could be a pituitary mass, the physician requests a full anterior pituitary hormone panel, and an MRI, demonstrated below.

Prolactin	35,000mU/L (Ref: 45-400mU/L)
Testosterone	3.5nmol/L (Ref: 10-27nmol/L)
FSH	5U/L (Ref: 2-11U/L)
LH	3U/L (Ref: 2-8U/L)
IGF-1	20nmol/L (Ref: 6-24nmol/L)
9AM Cortisol	650nmol/L (Ref: 150-650nmol/L)
MRI Pituitary Non-Contrast:	4cm Pituitary Mass, with 2cm suprasellar invasion Impinging upon Optic Chiasm

Which of the following is the most likely diagnosis?

a) Macroprolactinoma
b) Pituitary Metastasis
c) Giant Prolactinoma
d) Pituitary Carcinoma
e) Collision Tumour

#82. All of the following are stimuli for the release of prolactin except:
- a) Shingles
- b) Nipple Rings
- c) Suckling
- d) Hypothyroidism
- e) Breast Examination
- f) All of the above will increase the release of prolactin

#83. 25-year-old female with a background of Hebephrenic Schizophrenia is referred to the Endocrine Department due to the demonstration of galactorrhoea. Her past medical history is significant for multiple antipsychotic medications, and a current serum prolactin measurement returns elevated at 2,000mU/L. Which of the following antipsychotic is the patient most likely prescribed?
- a) Clozapine
- b) Olanzapine
- c) Quetiapine
- d) Risperidone

#84. The management of medication-induced hyperprolactinaemia is guided by the symptomatology, and not the serum prolactin levels. Which of the following are viable options to manage the patient in question #83?
- a) Withhold the medication under psychiatric supervision and retest the serum prolactin levels in three days
- b) Continue medication under observation if asymptomatic
- c) If applicable, change to a prolactin-sparing antipsychotic (risking relapse and weight gain)
- d) Add oestrogen if cannot change medication (to prevent galactorrhoea and long-term complications such as hypogonadism and osteopaenia)
- e) Addition of a dopamine agonist (risking worsening psychiatric symptoms)
- f) Attempt to decrease the current dosage of antipsychotic to reduce prolactin levels
- g) Add Aripiprazole
- h) All of the above

#85. Thyroid hormones (T3 and T4) act through negative feedback in the pituitary gland to decrease the release of TSH and maintain homeostasis. Which of the following pituitary receptors do the thyroid hormones act upon to inhibit TSH?

       a)   Thyroid-Receptor Beta-1
       b)   Thyroid-Receptor Alpha-1
       c)   Thyroid-Receptor Beta-2
       d)   Thyroid-Receptor Alpha-2

#86. Chronic corticosteroid administration decreases the release of TSH, and which of the other following anterior pituitary hormones?

       a)   Prolactin
       b)   LH and FSH
       c)   GH
       d)   b) and c)
       e)   a) and c)

#87. Which of the following are predictors for an increased risk of developing hyperprolactinaemia with commencement of antipsychotic medication?

       a) D_2 receptor mutation (TaqIA Aq & A0241G)
       b)   Male
       c)   Elderly
       d)   Typical Antipsychotic
       e)   a) and b)
       f)   a) and d)

#88. Which of the following Endocrinological Disorders best characterises the following description: *"Prolonged Anovulation, Galactorrhoea and Amenorrhoea for greater than six months post-partum in a mother who is not nursing the infant. The absence of menstruation may lead to uterine atrophy. May resolve completely."*

       a)   Lymphocytic Hypophysitis
       b)   Sheehan's Syndrome
       c)   Chiari-Frommel Syndrome
       d)   Forbes-Albright Syndrome
       e)   Ahumada-del Castillo Syndrome

#89. Which of the following best characterises a macroprolactinoma occurring as a result of a familial syndrome, such as Multiple Endocrine Neoplasia?

a) More likely to be clinically silent
b) More likely to respond to treatment
c) More likely to be aggressive
d) More likely to not respond to treatment
e) a) and b)
f) b) and c)
g) c) and d)

#90. Although extremely uncommon, with only a couple hundred cases documented, pituitary carcinomas are known to be resistant to dopamine agonists, and radiotherapy. They are typically diagnosed after failure of these treatments. Which of the following alkylating agents has demonstrated promising results in the management of a pituitary carcinoma?

a) Temozolomide
b) Chlorambucil
c) Ifosfamide
d) Carboplatin
e) Melphalan

#91. Thyroid-Stimulating Hormone (TSH), upon binding to the TSH receptor, stimulates either the G_S (cAMP), or G_q pathway (IP/Calcium). Which of the following correctly pairs the G-protein pathway and its respective function?

a) G_s is responsible for hormone secretion, iodide uptake and glandular growth/differentiation
b) G_q mediates the rate-limiting pathway for the synthesis of thyroid hormones by iodide organification
c) G_s mediates the rate-limiting pathway for the synthesis of thyroid hormones by iodide organification
d) G_q is responsible for hormone secretion, iodide uptake and glandular growth/differentiation
e) a) and b)
f) c) and d)

#92. Ectopic ACTH Syndrome is notorious for demonstrating severe hypokalaemia and hyperpigmentation. Hypokalaemia is due to which of the following?

    a) Saturation of 11-Beta-Hydroxysteroid Dehydrogenase Type 1

    b) Stimulation of 11-Beta-Hydroxysteroid Dehydrogenase Type 1

    c) Saturation of 11-Beta-Hydroxysteroid Dehydrogenase Type 2

    d) Inhibition of 11-Beta-Hydroxysteroid Dehydrogenase Type 2

#93. With Giant Prolactinomas, many authors note a paradoxical rise in prolactin after testosterone replacement. Which of the following may explain this peculiarity?

    a) Testosterone increases the release of all anterior pituitary hormones

    b) Assay interference

    c) Testosterone is converted to oestrogen through the aromatase enzyme, which may increase the release of prolactin

    d) Testosterone increases levels of Thyroid-Stimulating Hormone (TSH), which is a stimulus for prolactin secretion

#94. Which of the following anterior pituitary hormones assists with the production of foetal surfactant?

    a) Prolactin

    b) TSH

    c) GH

    d) a-MSH

#95. All of the following are true regarding prolactin except for:

    a) Increased by opiates

    b) Increase at the climax of sexual intercourse

    c) Counteract the anti-inflammatory effects of glucocorticoids

    d) Shortens the luteal phase in women

    e) All of the above are correct

#96. Which hormone functions alongside prolactin to assist in the 'let-down' reflex during suckling?

- a) Cortisol
- b) Oxytocin
- c) Oestriol
- d) Oestradiol
- e) Androstenedione

#97. Which of the following classes of medications may result in Hypophysitis?

- a) CTLA-4 Immunotherapy
- b) Isoniazid
- c) Second-Generation Sulfonylureas
- d) Alkylating Agents
- e) Biguanides

#98. A 62-year-old female, three-months post traumatic brain injury, is brought to her general physician by her husband, who notes lethargy, tiredness and dryness of her skin. A thyroid hormone profile is performed, demonstrating secondary hypothyroidism. Which of the following is this patient likely to demonstrate on physical examination?

- a) Goitre
- b) Weight Gain
- c) Weight Loss
- d) Hot flushes
- e) c) and d)
- f) a) and d)

#99. Which of the following vitamins listed below characterises the following description: *"Both a concurrent deficit or elevation of this vitamin may lead to peripheral neuropathy. Moreover, this vitamin is known to inhibit the release of prolactin."*

- a) Vitamin B1 (Thiamine)
- b) Vitamin B3 (Niacin)
- c) Vitamin B6 (Pyridoxine)
- d) Vitamin B9 (Folic Acid)
- e) Vitamin B12 (Cyanocobalamin)

#100. Which of the following gut hormones is believed to be responsible for the transient rise in prolactin levels after a meal?
    a) Ghrelin
    b) Glucagon-Like-Peptide-1 (GLP-1)
    c) Gastric Inhibitory Polypeptide (GIP)
    d) Vasoactive Intestinal Peptide (VIP)
    e) Secretin

#101. Which of the following is co-released with vasopressin, and has been noted to stimulate the release of prolactin?
    a) Prolactin Releasing Peptide
    b) Copeptin
    c) Kisspeptin
    d) Neurophysin II

#102. Which two anterior pituitary hormones bind to transmembrane receptors, which interact through the Janus Kinase (JAK) pathway?
    a) Prolactin and ACTH
    b) ACTH and TSH
    c) FSH and LH
    d) ACTH and FSH/LH
    e) GH and Prolactin

#103. Prolactin acts via negative feedback in the central nervous system to secrete dopamine from the hypothalamus via induction of which of the following enzymes?
    a) Tyrosine Kinase
    b) DOPA Decarboxylase
    c) Tyrosine Hydroxylase
    d) Phenylalanine Hydroxylase

#104. The release of prolactin is pulsatile, with their levels highest during which stage of sleep?
    a) Stage 1 non-REM
    b) Stage 2 non-REM
    c) Stages 3 & 4, non-REM
    d) Rapid Eye Movement (REM) Sleep

#105. Oxytocin is cleaved from the peptide precursor coded by the OXT gene. The final hydrolysis for which oxytocin is released is due to

the enzyme Peptidylglycine alpha-amidating monooxygenase (PAM).
Which of the following is a necessary co-factor for this enzyme?

  a) Vitamin B6
  b) Vitamin C
  c) Vitamin A
  d) Iron
  e) Zinc

#106. Oxytocin is noted to be released following gastric distension, and may lead to a suppression of food intake. Which of the following gut hormones has been demonstrated to increase the release of oxytocin?

  a) Glucagon-Like-Peptide-1 (GLP-1)
  b) Cholecystokinin (CCK)
  c) Secretin
  d) Somatostatin
  e) Glucagon
  f) Gastrin

#107. Which of the following pituitary hormones shares structural similarities with the hormone vasopressin, and when used in excess may lead to hyponatraemia?

  a) Copeptin
  b) Oxytocin
  c) Neurophysin
  d) Prolactin
  e) TSH

#108. Which of the following correctly identifies the difference between Cerebral Salt-Wasting (CSW) and Syndrome of Inappropriate ADH (SIADH)?

  a) SIADH is Hypervolaemic; CSW is Euvolaemic
  b) SIADH is Euvolaemic; CSW is Hypervolaemic
  c) SIADH is Euvolaemic, CSW is Hypovolaemic
  d) SIADH is treated with saline administration; CSW is treated with fluid restriction
  e) SIADH is treated with fluid restriction; CSW is treated with saline administration
  f) a) and d)
  g) c) and e)

#109. A 62-year-old gentleman presents to his family physician with a three-year history of 'bone pains'. On further elaboration, the gentleman explains that his wedding ring no longer fits, and both wrists feel 'tight' with a tingling sensation in the digits. He was initially diagnosed as osteoarthritis two years ago; however, his symptoms have worsened, and he is concerned as he has recently been diagnosed with diabetes. The physician requests the following biochemical investigations:

Prolactin	400mU/L (Ref: 45-400mU/L)
Testosterone	10nmol/L (Ref: 10-27nmol/L)
FSH	5U/L (Ref: 2-11U/L)
LH	3U/L (Ref: 2-8U/L)
IGF-1	60nmol/L (Ref: 8-25nmol/L)
9AM Cortisol	620nmol/L (Ref: 150-650nmol/L)

Which of the following is the most likely diagnosis?
- a) Acromegaly
- b) Cushing's Disease
- c) Gigantism
- d) Cushing's Syndrome
- e) Hyperthyrotrophinoma

#110. Which of the following imaging modalities is the first step towards investigation of the disorder characterised in question #109?
- a) CT with contrast
- b) MRI non-contrast with 2mm slices
- c) MRI with contrast with 2mm slices
- d) CT non-contrast

#111. Which of the following is the paediatric counterpart to Acromegaly?
- a) Acromegaloidism
- b) Sotos Syndrome
- c) Beckwith-Wiedemann Syndrome
- d) Gigantaloidism
- e) Gigantism

#112. The anterior pituitary hormone co-released with Growth Hormone in up to 30% of cases of Acromegaly is:
- a) TSH
- b) Prolactin
- c) Somatostatin

d)   ACTH

<u>#113.</u> From the onset of symptoms, the diagnosis of acromegaly is on average diagnosed after how many years?
       a)   One to Five Years
       b)   Five to Ten Years
       c)   Twenty + Years

<u>#114.</u> Cushing's' Disease is most commonly due to a microadenoma. What percentage of Acromegaly is due to a pituitary adenoma?
       a)   25%
       b)   45%
       c)   65%
       d)   85%
       e)   95%

<u>#115.</u> Which of the following dietary factors are known to increase the levels of Insulin-Like-Growth Factor 1 (IGF-1)?
       a)   Dairy
       b)   Protein
       c)   Glucose
       d)   All of the above

<u>#116.</u> A 72-year-old gentleman is diagnosed with acromegaly after a six-year history of coarsening facial features, loss of peripheral vision and diabetes-related complications. An MRI contrast of the pituitary denoted a 1.5cm macroadenoma. Prior to a transsphenoidal resection, the IGF-1 serum level was 87nmol/L (Ref: 18-36nmol/L). At eight weeks postoperative, an anterior pituitary hormone panel is performed, demonstrated below:

Oral Glucose Tolerance Test	GH Nadir Concentration: 1.8micrograms/L
IGF-1	50nmol/L (Ref: 7-24nmol/L)
Synthetic ACTH Stimulation Cortisol	650nmol/L (Ref: > 450nmol/L)
Free T4	10pmol/L (Ref: 8-22pmol/L)
TSH	2mU/L (Ref: 0.5-4.5mU/L)
Prolactin	300mU/L (Ref: 45-400mU/L)
MRI Contrast	No residual tissue identified

Which of the following is the likely diagnosis?
       a)   Inadequate resection of the adenoma
       b)   Permanent Hypopituitarism
       c)   Adequate resection

d) Cannot be determined at eight weeks postoperatively

#117. A 58-year-old female with a clinical phenotype suspicious for Acromegaly is referred to the endocrinologist for further investigation. She has a 4-year-history of worsening, irretractable headaches, carpal tunnel syndrome (bilateral), arthralgia, hypertension, sleep apnoea and prognathism. The physician performs an IGF-1 serum sample and an MRI of the head, with the results demonstrated below.

IGF-1	42nmol/L (Ref: 9-25nmol/L)
MRI Head Contrast	Sella turcica filled with cerebrospinal fluid, limited pituitary tissue visualised.

Which of the following is the likely diagnosis?

a) Paraneoplastic Growth Hormone Release
b) Ectopic Growth Hormone-Releasing Hormone Release
c) Hypothalamic Ganglioneuroma (hypersecretion of Growth Hormone Releasing Hormone)
d) Pituitary Adenoma (Empty Sella Syndrome)
e) Falsely elevated IGF-1

#118. Insulin-Like-Growth Factor 1 (IGF-1), also known as Somatomedin C, is the primary screening test for diagnosing Acromegaly. All of the following options listed below may increase the IGF-1 except for:

a) Pregnancy
b) Adolescence
c) Diabetes Mellitus
d) Oral Oestrogen
e) Postoperative (short-term)
f) Hyperthyroidism
g) Levothyroxine replacement for Hypothyroidism
h) Short-term Corticosteroid Usage
i) IGF-1 Receptor Mutation

#119. IGF-1 serum levels must be correctly correlated to the patient's Age, Gender and Body Mass Index. Which of the following options correctly suggests what happens to IGF-1 and GH with increasing age?

a) IGF-1 levels do not change; GH levels decrease
b) IGF-1 levels increase; GH levels do not change
c) IGF-1 levels decrease; GH levels increase

d) IGF-1 levels decrease; GH levels decrease
e) IGF-1 levels increase; GH levels increase

#120. An Oral Glucose Tolerance may be performed when IGF-levels are equivocal. This is done with the administration of 75 grammes of oral glucose, and serum GH measurement two hours later. A value greater than which of the following options is diagnostic for Acromegaly?
a) 2.5ng/mL
b) 1.5ng/mL
c) 1.0ng/mL
d) 0.5ng/mL
e) 0.4ng/mL

#121. Which of the following options may lead to a lowered IGF-1 serum level?
a) Hypothyroidism
b) Malnutrition
c) Type 1 Diabetes Mellitus (Poor Control)
d) Liver Failure
e) Renal Failure
f) All of the above

#122. Growth Hormone hypersecretion may lead to all of the following biochemical results, except for:
a) Hypercalciuria
b) Hypophosphataemia
c) Hypercalcaemia
d) Hypertriglyceridaemia
e) Hyperglycaemia

#123. Which of the following cancers are present at an increased prevalence in patients with acromegaly?
a) Thyroid Cancer
b) Colorectal Cancer
c) Stomach
d) Melanoma
e) All of the above

#124. Patients with acromegaly on average have a 10-year reduction in lifespan compared to the general population (72% increased mortality). Which of the following is the commonest cause of mortality for these patients?

        a)   Malignancy
        b)   Diabetes Mellitus
        c)   Respiratory Dysfunction (Sleep Apnoea)
        d)   Cardiovascular Disease

#125. It is recommended that the measurement of IGF-1 is performed either in patients with typical acromegalic manifestations or known associated conditions. Which of the following represents an 'active symptom' of acromegaly?

        a)   Sweating
        b)   Hypertension
        c)   Diastema
        d)   Increased shoe size
        e)   a) and b)
        f)   a) and d)

#126. Following a successful transsphenoidal surgical resection of a growth-hormone secreting macroadenoma, a 64-year-old female would like to know which symptoms may persist. Which of the following symptoms may persistent after successful resection?

        a)   Sleep Apnoea
        b)   Arthralgia
        c)   Valvulopathy
        d)   Diabetes Mellitus
        e)   Hyperhidrosis
        f)   a), b) c) and d)
        g)   a), b) and c)
        h)   a), c) and e)

#127. A false-positive Growth Hormone suppression may occur in all but which of the following situations?

        a)   Liver Failure
        b)   Renal Failure
        c)   Adolescence
        d)   Malnutrition/Anorexia Nervosa
        e)   All of the above may cause false positives

#128. Which of the following may lead to a paradoxical increase in GH after the glucose tolerance test?

a) Thalassaemia
b) Diabetes Mellitus
c) Alcohol Intoxication
d) Aspirin administration
e) None of the above

#129. Which of the following additional surgeries should be considered following a successful transsphenoidal resection of a pituitary macroadenoma (with undetectable IGF-1 and GH post-operatively after twelve weeks)?
a) Uvolopalatopharyngoplasty
b) Bowel Resection
c) Maxillofacial Reconstruction
d) Thyroidectomy
e) Tonsillectomy
f) Joint Replacement

#130. A 62-year-old gentleman patient undergoes a transsphenoidal resection of a macroadenoma for biochemical and radiological confirmed Acromegaly. Twelve weeks later, she is followed-up for assessment of remission, with the following results:

IGF-1	100nmol/L (Ref: 7-24nmol/L).
MRI Head Contrast	Residual Tissue extending towards the cavernous sinus

A multi-disciplinary team concludes that the patient is not a candidate for a re-operation due to the invasion of the cavernous sinus. It is explained to the patient that he will not be suitable for another repeat surgery but will be managed with a somatostatin ligand (Octreotide). The gentleman is furious at the 'incompetent' surgeons and is considering filing a lawsuit for negligence. The physicians should explain:
a) The surgery made no difference; he will have the same response to Octreotide whether or not a resection took place
b) The incomplete surgery will make the residual tissue resistant to the effects of octreotide
c) The incomplete surgery will make the residual tissue more sensitive to octreotide ('debulking)
d) Whilst microadenomas are cured with surgery in up to 90% of cases, only around 50% of macroadenomas are cured with surgery

e) a) and d)
f) b) and d)
g) c) and d)

#131. Following successful transsphenoidal resection of a macroadenoma, a patient treated for acromegaly would like to know up to how long can it take for reversal of his visual field deficits?

a) 24 Hours
b) One Week
c) One Month
d) One Year

#132. The initial treatment modality for both pituitary and ectopic Acromegaly is:

a) IGF-1 Receptor Antagonist
b) Somatostatin Receptor Ligand
c) Dopamine Agonist
d) Surgery
e) Radiotherapy

#133. Following an unsuccessful resection of a pituitary macroadenoma (acromegaly), a 72-year-old female is to be commenced upon medication for the management of the residual tumourous tissue. The following options are explained to her:

Significant Residual Disease Post-Resection	Somatostatin receptor ligand or pegvisomant
Modest IGF-1 Elevation & mild signs of Acromegaly	Trial of cabergoline
Inadequate response to somatostatin receptor ligand	Combine somatostatin receptor ligand with either pegvisomant or cabergoline

The patient is commenced upon Octreotide Injection. Which of the following is a potential complication of Octreotide for which the patient must be warned of?

a) Gallstones
b) Worsening headaches
c) Hypoglycaemia
d) Tachycardia
e) Diarrhoea

#134. Which of the following medications used in the management of acromegaly significantly worsens the hyperglycaemia index?

164

a) Pasireotide
b) Octreotide
c) Pegvisomant
d) Cabergoline

#135. Which of the following options correctly distinguishes
Somatostatin Receptor Ligands from Pegvisomant?
a) Somatostatin Receptor Ligands normalise IGF-1
levels in up to 90% with no effect upon tumour
size. Pegvisomant decreases IGF-1 levels in 60%
and reduces tumour size in ~50%.
b) Somatostatin Receptor Ligands normalise IGF-1
levels in up to 60% and reduce tumour size in
~50%. Pegvisomant decreases IGF-1 levels in
around 90% and reduces tumour size in virtually
all patients.
c) Somatostatin Receptor Ligands and
Pegvisomant are equally effective in serum IGF-
1 reduction and shrinkage of tumour
d) Somatostatin Receptor Ligands normalise IGF-1
levels in up to 60% and reduce tumour size in
~50%. Pegvisomant decreases IGF-1 levels in
around 90% but may increase tumour size.

#136. In which of the following patients is 'Iatrogenic Acromegaly' a
potential concern?
a) Turner's Syndrome
b) Soto's Syndrome
c) Marfan's Syndrome
d) Wilson's Syndrome
e) Menke's Kinky Hair Syndrome

#137. Growth-Hormone Secreting Macroadenomas, the commonest
cause of Acromegaly, may be further subdivided into two categories.
Which of the following options is correct regarding the two subtypes?
a) Densely Granulated (less responsive to
somatostatin receptor ligands); Sparsely
Granulated (more responsive to somatostatin
receptor ligands)

b) Densely Granulated and Perinuclear Granulated (equally responsive to somatostatin receptor ligands)
c) Perinuclear Granulated and Sparsely Granulated (equally responsive to somatostatin receptor ligands)
d) Densely Granulated (more responsive to somatostatin receptor ligands); Sparsely Granulated (less responsive to somatostatin receptor ligands)

<u>#138.</u> A 64-year-old gentleman attends follow-up appointment with his Endocrinologist. Six months ago, he underwent a transsphenoidal resection of an adenoma for Acromegaly, which was unsuccessful. Due to residual disease, he was commenced upon injectable medication. Despite full adherence to the medication, he has complained of worsening vision, and has had to recently give up driving. The Endocrinologist requests a hormonal panel to determine the efficacy of the medication, which is shown below.

Oral Glucose Tolerance Test	GH Nadir Concentration: 5.0micrograms/L
IGF-1	12nmol/L (Ref: 18-35nmol/L)
MRI Contrast Head	Compared to MRI 6/12, adenoma has enlarged and is encroaching upon optic chiasm

Which of the following is the most likely explanation?
a) Poor adherence
b) Resistance to Medication
c) Recurrence of disease
d) Infrequent, but expected side-effect of the medication

<u>#139.</u> Which of the following are further side-effects of the medication the patient is likely taking in question #138?
a) Lipohypertrophy
b) Lipoatrophy
c) Elevated Liver-Function Tests
d) Worsening Glycaemia
e) a), b) and c)
f) a), b) and d)
g) a), b), c) and d)

#140. Should neither surgical resection, nor medication therapy treat an underlying adenoma causing Acromegaly, radiotherapy is considered the 'third line' option. It is performed with adjuvant medication, as it has a slow effect (up to ten years). Annual GH/IGF-1 monitoring post medication withdrawal; periodic three-monthly medication withdrawals may be performed to measure GH and IGF-1. Which of the following is true regarding stereotactic radiotherapy?

    a) Lower risk of hypopituitarism
    b) Shorter duration of treatment
    c) Shortened time to remission
    d) Decreased Cognitive Decline
    e) All of the above
    f) None of the above

#141. Hypopituitarism may occur in up to how many percentages of patients treated with radiotherapy over the subsequent five-to-ten years?

    a) 10%
    b) 30%
    c) 50%
    d) 90%

#142. 'Skin Tags' are seen in states of insulin resistance, such as type 2 diabetes mellitus, cushing's syndrome, pregnancy and acromegaly. Which of the following is the correct medical term for 'skin tags'?

    a) Pseudosarcomatous Polyp
    b) Acrochordon
    c) Pinkus Tumour
    d) Seborrhoeic Keratosis

#143. Ectopic ACTH Syndrome, responsible for up to 20% of cases of Cushing's Syndrome, is more common amongst elderly males with a smoking history. Occasionally, Octreotide Scintigraphy can be used to detect these neuroendocrine tumours (which express somatostatin receptors 2 and 5). Which of the following may lead to a false positive with octreotide scanning?

    a) Fibrosis
    b) Inflammation
    c) Accessory spleen
    d) Breast Cancer
    e) Lymphoma

f) All of the above
g) b), c) and d)

#144.
#144. A 68-year-old retired professor is under investigation for Acromegaly, as denoted by the phenotypical manifestations of diastema, prognathism, hyperhidrosis, severe (bilateral) carpal tunnel syndrome and a thyroid goitre. Upon screening, the IGF-1 serum level is returned elevated at 56nmol/L (Ref: 6-24nmol/L). MRI of the pituitary, however, denotes no adenoma. The physician requests the additional investigation of GHRH, which returns elevated. Which of the following is the commonest location for ectopic acromegaly?

a) Phaeochromocytoma
b) Medullary Thyroid Carcinoma
c) Bronchial Carcinoid
d) Lymphoma

#145. A 54-year-old child-minder presents to her family physician due to the concern she is 'looking like Frankenstein'. She has noted a massive enlargement in her hands, jaw and neck. Moreover, she is beginning to note tingling sensations in her wrists and ankles. Upon reading various discussions forums online, she is concerned she has a condition known as 'Acromegaly', to which the physician agrees. The biochemical results are demonstrated below.

IGF-1	19nmol/L (Ref: 10-28nmol/L)
Oral Glucose Tolerance Test	GH Nadir Concentration: 0.2micrograms/L
Growth Hormone Releasing Hormone	20pg/mL (Ref: <49pg/mL)
MRI Head Contrast	Pituitary visualised, no abnormality/adenoma noted
Chest, Abdomen and Pelvis CT	Unremarkable

The physician, rather confused, refers this lady to an endocrinologist. Assuming the above test results are the true values (no laboratory error), which of the following is the likely diagnosis?

a) Acromegaloidism
b) Paget's Disease
c) Pachydermoperiostosis
d) Ectopic Acromegaly
e) Body Dysmorphic Disorder

#146. The diagnosis in question #145 is believed to be a result of increased levels of which of the following?

a) Somatostatin
b) Growth Factor
c) IGF-Binding Protein-3 (IGFBP-3)
d) Human Chorionic Somatomammotrophin

#147. In which of the following situations will stereotactic radiotherapy (compared to conventional radiotherapy) not be appropriate?

a) Residual Densely Granulated Tissue Subtype
b) Residual Sparsely Granulated Tissue Subtype
c) Residual tissue near optic chiasm
d) a) and c)
e) b) and c)

#148. A static acromegalic phenotype believed to occur as a result of an infarcted GH adenoma is referred to as:

a) Resistant Acromegaly
b) Burned Out Acromegaly
c) Pseudoacromegaly
d) Acromegaloidism

#149. Which of the following options may lead to 'pseudoacromegaly' (Acromegaloid appearance)?

a) Chronic Phenytoin Administration
b) Chronic, Severe Hypothyroidism
c) Chronic Minoxidil Administration
d) Type A Insulin Resistance
e) Ascher's Syndrome
f) All of the above
g) a) and c)

#150. A 61-year-old female patient attends the clinic with the complaint of headaches, joint stiffness and arthralgia. On Examination, it is notable that the patient has difficulty hearing, in addition to enlarged bones of the skull and prognathism (protruded jaw). Previous images over the past two years are given to the physician, who notes quite a distinction between her previous and current state. A diagnosis of Acromegaly is contemplated with her blood results demonstrated below.

IGF-1	16nmol/L (Ref: 8-23nmol/L)
Oral Glucose Tolerance Test	GH Nadir Concentration:

	0.3micrograms/L
Growth Hormone Releasing Hormone	22pg/mL (Ref: <49pg/mL)
MRI Head Contrast	Unremarkable
Chest, Abdomen and Pelvis CT	Unremarkable

The physician phones the laboratory to ask for an add-on test, measuring alkaline phosphate, calcium and parathyroid hormone levels. Which of the following options is the physician contemplating?

a) Multiple Myeloma
b) Paget's Disease
c) Cushing's Syndrome
d) Hyperparathyroidism-Jaw-Tumour Syndrome
e) Osteopetrosis

#151. Which of the following hormones are measured during an insulin-stress test?

a) Glucagon
b) Cortisol
c) Prolactin
d) Growth Hormone
e) IGF-1
f) b), c) and d)
g) a), c) and d)

#152. A 44-year-old female presents to the family physician with a three-year history of amenorrhoea and 'hot flushes'. Her physical examination is unremarkable, with no visual deficits perceived. A breast examination is negative for galactorrhoea on expression. A full hormonal profile is demonstrated below.

IGF-1	8nmol/L (Ref: 11-30nmol/L)
Prolactin	400mU/L (Ref: 60-620mU/L)
Oestradiol	40pmol/L (Ref: 200-2,000pmol/L)
FSH	1.6U/L (Ref: 3-11U/L)
LH	0.4U/L (Ref: 2-8U/L)
Free T4	15pmol/L (Ref: 10-22pmol/L)
TSH	<0.1mU/L (Ref: 0.37-5mU/L)
MRI Contrast Head	1.4x1.3cm mass, with no immediate concern for impingement upon optic chiasm

The physician decides to pursue an insulin-stress test:

Time (Minutes)	0	30	45	60	90	120
Glucose (mmol/L)	5.1	1.5	2.3	2.4	2.9	3.6
Cortisol (nmol/L)	415	412	580	560	480	400
GH (mU/L)	0.4	0.2	0.3	0.2	0.2	<0.1

What is the most likely diagnosis?

a) Sufficient Growth Hormone Reserve
b) Growth Hormone Deficiency
c) ACTH Deficiency
d) Combined ACTH and Growth Hormone Deficiency

#153. Although considered the 'Gold Standard' for diagnosing Growth Hormone Deficiency, an Insulin Tolerance Test lacks reproducibility, which is a significant disadvantage. Which of the following options listed is **not** a contraindication to perform the Insulin Tolerance Test?

a) Ischaemic Heart Disease
b) Epilepsy
c) Untreated Hypothyroidism
d) Untreated Hypoadrenalism
e) Pregnancy
f) Elderly (Above age 65)
g) History of Cerebrovascular and/or Coronary Artery Disease
h) Metabolic disorders such as glycogen storage Disease
i) All of the above are contraindications

#154. Why must hypothyroidism be treated prior to performing an insulin tolerance test?

a) Hypothyroidism falsely increases GH and IGF-1
b) Hypothyroidism impairs the release of Growth Hormone
c) Hypothyroidism falsely increases cortisol levels
d) Hypothyroidism impairs the release of cortisol
e) b) and c)
f) b) and d)

#155. A 44-year-old male presents to his general practitioner with worsening weight gain, fatigue and lethargy. His background medical history is significant for cranial irradiation as a child for leukaemia, which was cured. An insulin tolerance test is performed below after an anterior pituitary panel returns equivocal.

Time (Minutes)	0	30	45	60	90	120
Glucose (mmol/L)	5.4	2.6	2.8	3.1	3.7	3.9
GH (mU/L)	1.4	1.4	0.9	0.4	0.2	<0.1
Cortisol (nmol/L)	350	450	520	580	500	350

Which of the following is the correct interpretation of this test?
          a)   Adult Growth Hormone Deficiency
          b)   Cannot be interpreted
          c)   Secondary Hypoadrenalism
          d)   Adequate Growth Hormone Reserve

#156. During an Insulin Tolerance Test, a failure of growth hormone to rise above which level suggests Adult Growth Hormone Deficiency?
          a)   3 micrograms/L
          b)   3.5 micrograms/L
          c)   4 micrograms/L
          d)   4.5 micrograms/L
          e)   5 micrograms/L

#157. Although the Gold Standard for diagnosing Growth Hormone Deficiency is the Insulin Tolerance Test, there are many drawbacks such as the potential danger of inducing hypoglycaemia, patient discomfort and constant supervision by a clinician required (with 50% dextrose in a syringe to reverse hypoglycaemia). Moreover, patients must constantly be vigilant and reports symptoms (may require IV antiemetics). Which of the following are additional tests available to assess for growth hormone deficiency in adults?
          a)   Macimorelin Stimulation Test
          b)   Glucagon Stimulation Test
          c)   Arginine-GHRH Test
          d)   All of the above
          e)   None of the above

#158. A 42-year-old woman is under the care of an endocrinologist for a potential case of growth hormone deficiency. Two years ago, she suffered a traumatic brain injury after an automobile accident, where she stayed in the ITU for three months. Her only significant medical history is asthma, for which she is prescribed an inhaler (not used in the last seven years), and the oral contraceptive pill as she is in a relationship with a long-term boyfriend. The physician would like to assess both for Growth Hormone and ACTH Deficiency. How long must the oral oestrogen be stopped for, and why?
          a)   Two days; falsely elevates GH levels
          b)   Two weeks; falsely decreases GH levels
          c)   Four weeks; suppresses both GH and cortisol
               release

d) Six days; falsely decreases cortisol levels
e) Six weeks; falsely increases cortisol levels

#159. Standard recommendations are to re-assess a patient's ACTH reserve after the initiation of Growth Hormone, as a deficiency may mask mild adrenal insufficiency. Which of the following anterior pituitary reserves should also be assessed, as Growth Hormone replacement may deplete the respective hormonal levels?
a) FSH/LH
b) TSH/Free T4
c) Prolactin
d) ADH

#160. Upon commencement of Growth Hormone replacement therapy, IGF-1 serum levels are monitored for an adequate response along with physical and historical findings. The IGF-1 level is to be checked two months after initiation, and may be increased by one or two micrograms, with IGF-1 tested every two months until IGF-1 target level is reached, then semi/annually. Which of the following is **not** a side effect of initiating growth hormone?
a) Peripheral Oedema
b) Myalgia, Arthralgia and Paraesthesia
c) Sleep Apnoea
d) Pseudotumour Cerebri
e) Macular Oedema and Proliferative Retinopathy
f) Scoliosis Progression
g) Slipped Capital Femoral Epiphysis
h) All of the above are potential complications

#161. For which of the following patients will an increased dosage of Growth Hormone be required?
a) Obesity
b) Transdermal oestrogen
c) Post-menopausal women
d) Laron-Type Dwarfism
e) Pregnancy and Lactation
f) b) and c)

#162. Growth Hormone Replacement therapy is contraindicated in which of the following situations except for:
a) Active Malignancy

b) Critically Ill
c) Acute respiratory failure
d) Pregnancy
e) Lactation
f) Growth Hormone Hypersensitivity
g) Prescription for Anti-Ageing
h) Under 18 years of age

#163. Although no longer a concern, in the primitive phases of growth hormone replacement therapy, cadaveric growth hormone was used (nowadays synthetic Growth Hormone is used). This led to the potential for contamination and death from which of the following disorders?

a) HIV
b) Tuberculosis
c) Hepatitis C
d) Creutzfeldt-Jakob Disease
e) Syphilis

#164. All of the following are benefits with prescribing growth hormone replacement therapy except for:

a) Improved Quality of Life
b) Increased Bone Mineral Density
c) Improved Body Composition (Increased Lipolysis, Decreased total body fat)
d) Decreased Insulin Resistance
e) Improvement in lipid profile

#165. Following a diagnosis of Growth Hormone Deficiency, the QoL-AGHDA (Quality of Life Assessment of Growth Hormone Deficiency in Adults) is performed. A score of at least 11 with the QoL-AGHDA in addition to already requiring hormonal replacement for other anterior pituitary hormones and a 'severe' growth hormone deficiency are the steps patients are suggested to follow to attain growth hormone replacement therapy. Which of the following describes 'severe' GH deficiency?

a) Peak GH Response below 5.0micrograms/L (ITT)
b) Peak GH Response below 4.0micrograms/L (ITT)
c) Peak GH Response below 3.5micrograms/L (ITT)
d) Peak GH Response below 3.0micrograms/L (ITT)
e) Peak GH Response below 2.0micrograms/L (ITT)

#166. There is no 'time limit' for growth hormone replacement in adults, and it can be continued indefinitely. National Institute for Health and Care Excellence (NICE; United Kingdom) Guidelines recommend reassessment after nine months of treatment, and to discontinue if QoL improvement is less than seven points. The QoL-AGHDA consists of 25 yes-or-no questions, divided into seven categories. Which of the following is **not** a category assessed in the QoL-AGHDA?

    a) Body Image and Distribution of Fat
    b) Energy Level
    c) Concentration and Libido
    d) Irritability and Temper
    e) Strength and Stamina
    f) Ability to Cope with Stress
    g) Physical and Mental Drive

#167. A 53-year-old male is referred to the endocrinology department for further investigation of arthralgia, perspiration and a goitre. A 75 two-hour oral glucose tolerance test is performed with the following findings:

Time (Minutes)	0	30	60	90	120
Glucose (mmol/L)	9	13	14.2	13.8	13.4
GH (mU/L)	12	17	32	41	29

A full anterior pituitary hormonal panel is performed, with the only significant result a prolactin level of 865mU/L (Ref: 45-400mU/L). Which of the following is the most cause for the elevated prolactin?

    a) Co-secretion with Growth Hormone
    b) Stalk Compression
    c) Macroprolactin
    d) Prolactinoma

#168. A 25-year-old female presents to her family physician with a three-month history of amenorrhoea. She has further noted recurrent headaches. She was previously fit and well, with no prescribed medication. A prolactin measurement returns significantly elevated at 8,000 mU/L (Ref: 100-500mU/L). Which of the following is the most important initial investigation?

    a) MRI Head Contrast
    b) CT Head Non-Contrast

c)   Repeat Assay to rule out Macroprolactin
d)   Urinary Beta-hCG
e)   Thyroid Hormone Panel

#169. A 15-year-old female has been receiving Growth Hormone replacement (0.7mg Subcutaneous Injection) since nine-years of age due to the suspicion for growth hormone deficiency (idiopathic) due to unexplained short stature. Which of the following is the most appropriate initial investigation?

a)   Continue Growth Hormone into adulthood; consider dosage increase
b)   Repeat Insulin-Stress Test; likely to continue to require Growth Hormone replacement into adulthood
c)   Repeat Insulin-Stress Test; unlikely to require Growth Hormone by adulthood
d)   Anterior pituitary hormone profile to assess for hypopituitarism

#170. A 5-year-old child, with a background history of recurrent ear infections is referred to the paediatric endocrinology department for an urgent assessment. The child has a known history of hypogonadism and short stature, for which he is currently awaiting genetic test results. Physical examination is notable for bulging of the eyes (proptosis), and the patient is repeatedly asking his mother for water (unquenchable thirst). A head CT- demonstrates wide-spread osteolytic lesions. Which of the following is the most likely diagnosis?

a)   Sarcoidosis
b)   Langerhans Cell Histiocytosis
c)   Churg-Strauss Syndrome
d)   Tay-Sachs Disease

#171. All of the following medications may lead to drug-induced nephrogenic diabetes insipidus except for:

a)   Methoxyflurane
b)   Colchicine
c)   Demeclocycline
d)   Lithium
e)   Tolvaptan
f)   Citalopram

#172. A 24-year-old male with type 1 diabetes mellitus is brought to the emergency department by his fiancé, who found him on the kitchen floor vomiting and semi-conscious. The patient has had two previous visits to the emergency department in the past year for diabetic ketoacidosis due to non-compliance. Upon physical examination however, there is black eschar around his left orbit and nose, suggestive of Rhizopus spp. The gentleman is commenced upon intravenous Amphotericin B alongside DKA protocol and is scheduled for emergency resection of the necrotic tissue. Post-operatively, there are no complaints. Upon day five of his Amphotericin B, he is noted to repeatedly asks the nurses for help accessing the bathroom, whereby very dilute urine is produced. Despite keeping a good intake of fluids, he is constantly thirsty. Which of the following serum samples is likely to be present in this patient?

      a) Hyperkalaemia
      b) Hypokalaemia
      c) Hypomagnesaemia
      d) Hypercalcaemia
      e) Hypocalcaemia
      f) b) and c)
      g) b) and d)

#173. Which of the following medication classes must be stopped prior to a water deprivation test, due to its known ADH-potentiation?

      a) Antifungals
      b) Corticosteroids
      c) NSAIDs
      d) Tetracycline Antibiotics

#174. A 28-year-old female PhD. Candidate presents to her general practitioner with the complaint of increased thirst. She explains that she consumes around five litres of water (ongoing for the past four months). There was no precipitating event, and her past medical history is unremarkable. She consents to a water-deprivation test, of which the results are demonstrated below:

Time	Volume of Urine (mL)	Urine Osmolality (mOsm/Kg)	Plasma Osmolality (mOsm/Kg)	Weight (lbs.)
08:00	600mL	63		122.4
08:30			282	
11:00				122.2

11:30	325mL	212	282	
14:00				121.9
14:30			294	
15:00	145mL	348		121.5
15:30			296	
16:00	62mL	965		121.1

Which of the following is the most likely diagnosis?

a) Partial Nephrogenic Diabetes Insipidus
b) Partial Cranial Diabetes Insipidus
c) Psychogenic Polydipsia
d) Syndrome of Inappropriate ADH Release (SIADH)
e) Nephrogenic Diabetes Insipidus
f) Cranial Diabetes Insipidus

#175. Which of the following medications may be trialled in SIADH?

a) Tolvaptan
b) Mannitol
c) Lithium
d) Demeclocycline
e) a) and b)
f) a) and d)

#176. It is important to be aware that the term 'Primary Polydipsia' is preferred over 'Psychogenic', as it may not always be due to a psychological comorbidity. Primary Polydipsia may be (i) psychogenic, (ii) iatrogenic or (iii) Dipsogenic. Which of the following best characterises Dipsogenic Diabetes Insipidus?

a) Lesion within the posterior pituitary gland, loss of thirst sensation
b) Lesion within the renal osmoreceptors, heightened sensation of thirst
c) Lesion within the hypothalamus, loss of thirst sensation
d) Lesion within the hypothalamus, heightened thirst sensation
e) Lesion within the posterior pituitary gland, heightened of thirst sensation

#177. It is predicted that up to 20% of patients with schizophrenia of chronic nature harbour primary polydipsia, irrespective of the medications. The hyponatraemia as a result of the disorder may further worsen psychiatric symptomatology. Which of the following historical factors are suggestive of primary polydipsia over diabetes insipidus?

a) Nocturia
b) Waking up at night to drink water
c) Associated psychiatric disorder
d) a) and b)
e) b) and c)
f) a) and c)

#178. Which of the following correctly identifies the mechanism of action of Tolvaptan?

a) Urea-induced diuresis
b) Hyperglycaemia-induced diuresis
c) Vasopressin antagonist at V1 receptor
d) Vasopressin antagonist at V2 receptor

#179. A 22-year-old female is admitted to the emergency department after bystanders called the police. The history upon transfer to the hospital is that she was running nude throughout the town telling bystanders she has seen 'the light' and has a cure for HIV. Upon examination, she looks restless, and is hyperactive. She explains she has not slept in three days, as she has a deadline to finish her 'cure' and send it to the FDA. Her speech is very fast and pressured. It is deemed that she does not have capacity, and is commenced upon a medication prescribed for this disorder. Three months later upon follow-up, she complains of frequent urination and thirst; she is very concerned this could be diabetes, as her mother presented with similar symptoms prior to a diagnosis of Type 2 Diabetes Mellitus. A water-deprivation test is performed, demonstrated below (before and after vasopressin administration).

Time (Hour)	Volume of Urine (mL)	Urine Osmolality (mOsm/Kg)	Plasma Osmolality (mOsm/Kg)
08:00	600mL	210	
08:30			292
11:00			
11:30	500mL	208	300
14:00			
14:30			301
15:00	500mL	208	
15:30			310
16:00	325mL	210	
Vasopressin Administration:		Urine Osmolality 204mOsm/kg	

Which of the following is the most likely diagnosis?
a) Primary Polydipsia
b) Nephrogenic Diabetes Insipidus
c) Cranial Diabetes Insipidus
d) Partial Nephrogenic Diabetes Insipidus

#180. If the Urine Osmolality in question #179 were to increase above 800mOsm/Kg after desmopressin administration, which of the following would be the most likely diagnosis?
a) Primary Polydipsia
b) Nephrogenic Diabetes Insipidus
c) Cranial Diabetes Insipidus
d) Partial Cranial Diabetes Insipidus

#181. Which of the following street drugs must always be considered as a cause of 'excess thirst' in an adolescent/young adults?
a) PCP
b) Glue Sniffing
c) MDMA
d) Cannabis

#182. Sjögren's Syndrome is a well-known cause of 'dry mouth' (xerostomia) for which patients may require increased amounts of water, with resultant primary polydipsia. Which of the following classes of medications may lead to xerostomia?
a) Antiepileptics
b) Anticholinergics
c) Cholimimetics
d) MAO-Inhibitors

#183. A 62-year-old female presents to the emergency department with a severe, lancinating pain cross her lower left face which had occurred earlier this morning upon applying make-up. The pain lasted for no more than five seconds but felt as if she was being 'electrocuted' as is visibly in tears from the pain. This is not the first time this has presented, and she is very concerned that she will not be able to manage the pain. Upon introduction of pharmacotherapy, she experiences a massive improvement, and the pain has remitted. Over the next three weeks, she begins to demonstrate lethargy, malaise and confusion. Upon rising from the seat on the bus, she faints, and is brought back to the emergency department. The following results are obtained from the physician:

Standing Blood Pressure	90/62mmHg
Serum Sodium	122mmol/L (Ref: 135-145mmol/L)
Urine Osmolality	320mOsm/Kg
Urine Sodium	50mEq/L

Which of the following medications was most likely initiated?
- a) Carbimazole
- b) Carbamazepine
- c) Amitriptyline
- d) Lithium

#184. Renal Isothenuria (the inability to concentrate urine) is common amongst which of the following haematological disorders?
- a) Sickle Cell Trait
- b) G6PD Deficiency
- c) Alpha-Thalassaemia
- d) Warm Autoimmune Haemolytic Anaemia

#185. The MRI 'Bright Spot' is a normal finding in the posterior pituitary gland in 90% of individuals; this can occasionally be used to distinguish Primary Polydipsia from Diabetes Insipidus. Which of the following options is correct?
- a) The bright spot is absent in primary polydipsia, but retained in both cranial and nephrogenic diabetes insipidus
- b) The bright spot is absent in nephrogenic diabetes insipidus, but retained in both primary polydipsia and cranial diabetes insipidus
- c) The bright spot is retained in primary polydipsia and nephrogenic diabetes insipidus, but absent in cranial diabetes insipidus
- d) The bright spot is retained in primary polydipsia, but absent in both cranial and nephrogenic diabetes insipidus
- e) The bright spot is retained in nephrogenic diabetes insipidus, but absent in both cranial diabetes insipidus and primary polydipsia

#186. A 62-year-old woman is referred to the endocrinology department with a depressed mood, confusion and an unquenchable thirst with frequent urination. She has a prior history of a prolactinoma, which was successfully resected, and a family history of an insulinoma. Which of the following is the likely cause of the frequent urination?

a) Hyperparathyroidism; Cranial Diabetes Insipidus
b) Hypoparathyroidism; Nephrogenic Diabetes Insipidus
c) Hyperkalaemia; Nephrogenic Diabetes Insipidus
d) Hyperparathyroidism; Nephrogenic Diabetes Insipidus
e) Hyperkalaemia; Cranial Diabetes Insipidus

#187. A water-deprivation test must be terminated in which of the following scenarios?

a) Serum sodium rises to above 150mmol/L
b) Body weight reduction by more than three percent
c) Orthostatic symptoms
d) a) and b)
e) a), b) and c)

#188. Which of the following options correctly matches the organ of origin for 'Vasopressinase' and its resultant syndrome?

a) Posterior Pituitary Gland (by-product of ADH); little clinical effect
b) Juxtaglomerular Apparatus; Nephrogenic Diabetes Insipidus
c) Macula Densa; no significant clinical effect
d) Placenta; Gestational Diabetes Insipidus
e) Liver; Anti-epileptic induction of Vasopressin (partial diabetes insipidus)

#189. Which of the following options is correct regarding chronic polydipsia?

a) Serum osmolality will decrease upon water-deprivation
b) Urine osmolality will increase upon water-deprivation
c) Results are indistinguishable from nephrogenic diabetes insipidus
d) Response to desmopressin administration

<u>#190.</u> Which of the following correctly characterises 'Beer Potomania'?

    a) Hypernatraemia and increased renal excretion of free water in patients drinking excess alcohol and poor dietary intake

    b) Hyponatraemia and increased renal excretion of free water in patients drinking excess alcohol and poor dietary intake

    c) Hyponatraemia and decreased renal excretion of free water (serum dilution) in patients drinking excess alcohol and poor dietary intake

    d) Hypernatraemia and decreased renal excretion of free water in patients drinking excess alcohol and poor dietary intake

<u>#191.</u> All of the following options listed are demonstrated in 'Wolfram Syndrome' except for which of the following?

    a) Diabetes Mellitus
    b) Diabetes Insipidus
    c) Optic Atrophy
    d) Autosomal Dominant Inheritance
    e) WFS1 Gene Mutation

<u>#192.</u> A 67-year-old female with a background history of Type 2 Diabetes Mellitus (controlled with metformin, diet and exercise) is brought to the emergency department after a sudden-onset severe headache, vomiting, and an inability to look outwards to the right side (CN VI Palsy). On assessment, she has a Glasgow Coma Scale of 13/15, and is complaining of severe nausea. A CT-non-contrast is performed, which demonstrates a pituitary adenoma with intratumoural haemorrhage. A diagnosis of pituitary apoplexy is subsequently confirmed on MRI. Which of the following options concerning the diagnosis is incorrect?

    a) The majority of patients are diagnosed with a pituitary adenoma after the apoplectic episode

    b) GnRH, TRH, Insulin, Octreotide and Cabergoline increase the risk of pituitary apoplexy

    c) Up to 75% of the pituitary gland is likely to be damaged by the time hypopituitarism is evident

> d) Females develop pituitary apoplexy twice as often as males
> e) Horner's Syndrome is a potential complication
> f) Pituitary apoplexy can compress the internal carotid artery within the cavernous sinus, leading to cerebral infarction

#193. Pituitary apoplexy is most common in the fifth-sixth decade of life, and most common with macroadenomas. The most common underlying adenoma with pituitary apoplexy is:

> a) Non-functioning adenoma
> b) GH Adenoma
> c) Prolactinoma
> d) TSHoma

#194. Asymptomatic apoplexy, further referred to as subclinical apoplexy, is more common than true pituitary apoplexy, occurring in around 20% of patients with a pituitary macroadenoma. Which of the following is correct regarding subclinical apoplexy?

> a) More common in females
> b) Most common with prolactinomas
> c) Occasionally of benefit; hypersecreting tumours may outgrow their blood supply leading to autohypophysectomy
> d) All of the above are correct
> e) a) and c)

#195. With pituitary apoplexy, up to 80% of patients will develop hormonal deficiencies. Which of the following is the most important axis to measure?

> a) Hypothalamo-pituitary-thyroid axis
> b) Hypothalamo-pituitary-adrenal axis
> c) Hypothalamo-pituitary-gonadal axis
> d) Hypothalamo-pituitary-hepatic (IGF-1) axis

#196. A 17-year-old girl presents to the physician with her mother, who is concerned that her daughter has not yet had her first menstrual cycle. The patient has two older sisters, both of whom began menstruating at age 13. On examination, the patient demonstrates secondary sexual characteristics within the pre-pubertal stage. The past medical history is unremarkable apart from a decreased sense of smell; however, it is evident that her hands 'mirror' each other when performing a movement. The mother says 'this is intentional', however the patient rather embarrassingly admits during class, whilst attempting to write with her right hand, the left hand performs the same movement. An anterior pituitary hormone profile is performed, of which, the results are demonstrated below:

Oestradiol	Decreased
FSH	Normal
LH	Normal
IGF-1	Normal

Which of the following is the most likely diagnosis?
- a) Congenital Isolated Hypogonadotrophic Hypogonadism
- b) Kallmann's Syndrome
- c) Non-functional Adenoma
- d) Pregnancy
- e) Lyme Disease

#197. A 22-year-old male college student makes an appointment with his family physician. In the past few weeks, he has failed to achieve an erection with his long-term girlfriend. Moreover, his sexual drive is diminished. He adamantly denies taking any 'legal or illegal' medications and asks for sildenafil to help with his erectile dysfunction. On examination, the gentleman has a muscular physique, and the physician notes bruising over his left antecubital fossa. Small testicles are noted on genital examination. A visual fields test is unremarkable. The following hormonal profiles are measured:

LH	Normal
FSH	Normal
Testosterone	Decreased
9AM Cortisol	Normal

Which of the following options correctly identifies the underlying diagnosis?
- a) Subclinical apoplexy
- b) Pituitary stalk impingement
- c) Macroprolactinoma
- d) Idiopathic hypogonadism
- e) Exogenous steroid administration

#198. Which of the following correctly characterises 'macroprolactin'?
- a) Only secreted by pituitary prolactinomas

    b) Indicator for malignancy
    c) Its presence suggests sensitivity to dopamine
       agonists
    d) Its presence refers to an inactive form
       conjugated to antibodies, being physiologically
       inert
    e) Characteristic of medication-induced
       hyperprolactinaemia

#199. Which of the options correctly defines the following description: *'Characterised by episodic hypersecretion of a hormone, with normal biochemical measurements in-between episodes. Postulated to occur as a result of haemorrhage into a pre-existing adenoma'*?

    a) Cyclic Cushing's Syndrome
    b) Burned-Out Acromegaly
    c) Intermittent Central Hyperthyroidism
    d) Periodic Hypergonadism

#200. Which of the following is the commonest cause of Cushing's Syndrome in pregnant females?

    a) Cushing's Disease
    b) Ectopic ACTH Syndrome
    c) Adrenal Adenoma
    d) Iatrogenic

#201. A 62-year-old gentleman presents to his GP with a three-month history of muscular weakness and weight gain. He has a 30-pack-year smoking history, and drinks three units of alcohol daily. On examination, oral thrush is noted, in addition to easy bruising and hyperpigmentation. The following results are obtained:

Urinary Free cortisol	862nmol/day (Ref: <300)
Low-dose dexamethasone suppression test	119nmol/L (Ref: <50)
ACTH	66ng/L (Ref: 10-50)
Potassium	3.2mmol/L (Ref: 3.5-5.3mmol/L)
High-Dose Dexamethasone Suppression Test	ABNORMAL
Chest X-ray	Left-perihilar, irregular 3x2cm mass, suspicious for malignancy

The gentleman is subsequently diagnosed with ectopic ACTH Syndrome. Which of the following is the most likely tumour subtype?

a) Squamous Cell Carcinoma
b) Adenocarcinoma
c) Small-Cell Lung Carcinoma
d) Adenocarcinoma
e) Large Cell Carcinoma

#202. Occasionally, ectopic ACTH syndrome is suppressed with the high-dose dexamethasone suppression test. Which of the following tumour subtypes may infrequently demonstrate this peculiarity (leading to diagnostic uncertainty)?
a) Adrenal Carcinoma
b) Phaeochromocytoma
c) Bronchial Carcinoid
d) Lymphoma

#203. Which of the following options correctly suggests why female patients with Cushing's Syndrome present with amenorrhoea?
a) ACTH functions as an antagonist at the ovarian follicle
b) Hyperandrogenaemia results in decreased FSH and LH release via negative feedback
c) Co-secretion of prolactin
d) Corticosteroids directly inhibit the responsiveness of GnRH, contributing to inhibition of the release of gonadotrophins

#204. All of the following medications may inhibit CYP3A4 (which metabolises dexamethasone) except for:
a) Fluoxetine
b) Ritonavir
c) Diltiazem
d) Cimetidine
e) Pioglitazone

#205. Which of the following situations will lead to a skewed urinary free cortisol measurement?
a) Urinary Tract Infection
b) Ingestion of large amounts of free water prior to and during collection
c) Creatinine Clearance below 60mL/min
d) Mild Cushing's Syndrome

e) All of the above

#206. Which of the following medications is prescribed in nephrogenic diabetes insipidus?
a) Hydrochlorothiazide
b) Spironolactone
c) Mannitol
d) Eplerenone
e) Furosemide

#207. de Morsier Syndrome (also known as septo-optic dysplasia) is a congenital malformation featuring underdevelopment of the pituitary gland, optic nerve and absent septum pellucidum (with two of the three present for diagnosis). Which of the following is the most common hormonal deficiency associated with this condition?
a) ACTH deficiency
b) GH deficiency
c) LH/FSH deficiency
d) TSH deficiency

#208. Midnight Salivary Cortisol levels may be falsely elevated in which of the following situations?
a) Night-shift workers
b) Ingestion of dairy products
c) Smoking/Licorice ingestion
d) High sugar or acid-containing foods
e) Hot drink/brushing teeth
f) All of the above

#209. A 31-year-old gentleman presents to his general practitioner with his wife. They have been trying to conceive for over two years now, without success. The wife has a previous daughter with her first husband, and the current husband has no children. The gentleman reports a slight decrease in libido, however, has attributed this to the stress of 'being a lawyer'. His pubertal history is unremarkable, as is his family history. In the last year, he has developed bilateral osteoarthritis of his hands, and was diagnosed as 'Prediabetic'. On examination, a mild tan is noticeable, in addition to bilateral decrease in testicular volume. An anterior pituitary profile is performed, with the results demonstrated below.

LH	3.1U/L (Ref: 2-8U/L)

FSH	7U/L (Ref: 2-11U/L)
Prolactin	306mU/L (Ref: 45-400mU/L)
8AM Testosterone	5nmol/L (Ref: 10-42nmol/L)
TSH	1.6mU/L (Ref: 0.37-5mU/L)
T4	18pmol/L (Ref: 10-22pmol/L)

The next most appropriate test in this patient is:
- a) Testicular Ultrasound
- b) Ferritin and iron saturation
- c) Brain MRI
- d) Caeruloplasmin measurement

#210. Which of the following investigations can be used to differentiate pseudo-cushing's disease from cushing's disease?
- a) Low-dose dexamethasone suppression test
- b) Dexamethasone-CRH test
- c) Insulin Stress Test
- d) All of the above

Pituitary Gland & Hypothalamus – Answers

<u>#1</u>. d) Oxytocin
The posterior pituitary gland stores both oxytocin and antidiuretic hormone (vasopressin), which are both synthesised within the hypothalamus. Prolactin, Growth Hormone, Follicle-Stimulating Hormone, Luteinising Hormone, ACTH and TSH are all released from the anterior pituitary gland.

<u>#2</u>. e) Supraoptic Nuclei (Vasopressin); Paraventricular Nuclei (Oxytocin)
Although significant overlap, Vasopressin is released in smaller amounts from the Paraventricular Nuclei, the latter of which being the main source for oxytocin.

<u>#3.</u> d) Cavernous Sinus
The Cavernous Sinus is located laterally to the pituitary gland, containing CN III, IV, V1, V2 and VI, in addition to the Internal Carotid Artery. Pituitary adenomas may expand and compress the structures within the cavernous sinus, leading to multiple clinical sequelae.

<u>#4.</u> d) Internal Carotid Artery
Superior hypophyseal artery supplies the hypothalamus and forms the hypophyseal portal circulation, which is in direct contact with the anterior pituitary gland. This functions to prevent systemic dilution of the releasing factors. This is a branch of the internal carotid artery.

<u>#5.</u> a) Meningohypophyseal Trunk
The inferior hypophyseal artery derives its blood supply from the meningohypophyseal trunk, which is the fourth segment of the internal carotid artery.

<u>#6.</u> a) Cushing's Disease
Inferior petrosal sinus sampling has largely replaced the large-dose dexamethasone suppression test as a diagnostic intervention for cushing's disease. ACTH is measured (bilaterally) within the inferior

petrosal sinus before and after corticotrophin-releasing hormone administration; a central-to-peripheral ratio of above 2.0 (before CRH administration) or >3.0 (after CRH administration) is diagnostic for pituitary-driven Cushing's Syndrome. Although infrequently encountered, false negatives do occur, particularly amongst improper catheter placement or anomalous venous drainage.

#7. b) Sheehan's Syndrome
The anterior pituitary gland nearly doubles in size during pregnancy and is at risk of ischaemic necrosis during post-partum haemorrhage. One of the first signs is the inability to lactate – it is important to be aware that most cases of hypopituitarism may present with hyperprolactinaemia (from pituitary stalk compression), but this is one of the rare conditions associated with hypoprolactinaemia.

#8. d) The posterior pituitary gland is unaffected as it functions under a high-pressure system
The posterior pituitary gland is relatively unaffected during Sheehan's Syndrome (postpartum haemorrhage). Whilst largely postulated, it is believed this is due to the posterior pituitary gland functioning under a higher-pressure system compared to its anterior counterpart. Moreover, as the hypothalamus synthesises the respective hormones, if the posterior pituitary gland is damaged, secretion may still be able to continue from the hypothalamus.

#9. c) Craniopharyngioma
A craniopharyngioma is a neoplastic growth of Rathke's Pouch remnants, and may present in children with diabetes insipidus, short stature, bitemporal hemianopia and headaches. Classically, it is identified as a supra-sellar calcification of neuroimaging.

#10. a) Seven Weeks
At around week six, cellular proliferation occurs within the anterior pituitary gland, and roughly one week afterward (week seven) primitive hormonal release is possible.

#11. e) 80%
The adenohypophysis (anterior pituitary gland) comprises the great majority of the pituitary gland (around 80%).

<u>#12.</u> c) Pars Inermedia
The Pars Intermedia (Intermediate Lobe) is formed from the posterior portion of the anterior pituitary gland. Although small, this lobe is believed to increase during pregnancy, and releases alpha-melanocyte-Stimulating Hormone.

<u>#13.</u> c) Melanocyte-Stimulating Hormone
The Intermediate Lobe, considered part of the anterior pituitary gland (posterior portion), has gained attention in recent years as it is believed to be able to release alpha-melanocyte stimulating hormone, and undergoes hypertrophy during gestation.

<u>#14.</u> b) Pars Nervosa
The Infundibulum gives rise to the pituitary stalk and the Pars Nervosa, (posterior pituitary gland).

<u>#15.</u> d) Somatotrophes
Somatotrophes (which release Growth Hormone) comprise 50% of anterior pituitary cells; therefore Growth Hormone is the first hormone to be lost in the hypopituitarism sequence. Lactotrophes comprise another 15%, as do Corticotrophes. Gonadotrophes constitute 10% and Thyrotrophes comprise the remaining 5%.

<u>#16.</u> a) Thyrotrophes
Thyrotrophes comprise around 5% of anterior pituitary cells and are the least numerous.

<u>#17.</u> e) Corticotrophes
Textbooks do vary; however, the author has most commonly encountered the following, which is in agreement with various references: GH > FSH/LH > TSH > ACTH. Prolactin is rarely decreased due to an adenoma, as it expands and compresses the pituitary stalk. This interrupts the dopamine-inhibition of prolactin, which therefore increases prolactin levels.

<u>#18.</u> d) Acidophil: Release Polypeptides; Basophils: Release Glycopeptides; Chromophobes: Do not release any hormone
Acidophil cells, constituting nearly 40% of the anterior pituitary cells, stain red with acidic dye. Acidophils release polypeptides (Growth Hormone and Prolactin). Basophil, constitute 10%, and stain blue with basic dyes. Basophils release Glycopeptides (LH, FSH, TSH, ACTH and b-

hCG). The reamining cells are known as Chromophobe cells, and do not
release any hormones; these are believed to be cells which previously
were either an acidophil or basophil, but have since lost their secretory
granules (and hence secretory function).

#19. e) Somatotrophes; Thyrotrophes
Somatotrophes are the most numerous anterior pituitary cells
(acidophils), whilst thyrotrophes are the least numerous anterior
pituitary cells (basophils).

#20. b) and c) (option e)
Prolactin-Inhibiting Hormone, also known as Dopamine, is released by
the hypothalamus and inhibits the release of prolactin. When there is
stalk interruption (such as with macroadenomas), dopamine fails to
reach lactotrophs and therefore levels are typically elevated.
Moreover, with antipsychotics and antiemetics functioning as
dopamine antagonists, prolactin levels will rise.

#21. c) Lactotrophes
Basophils release glycoproteins, which include FSH, LH, ACTH, TSH and
beta-hCG. Lactotrophes are acidophils (alongside somatotrophes),
which release polypeptides.

#22. d) Alpha subunit is the common ancestral subunit; Beta-subunit
functions to determine specificity
The beta-subunit confers the specificity of the glycoprotein, whereby
the alpha-subunit is common to all glycoproteins. This is important in
clinical situations such as Hyperemesis Gravidarum or Hypothyroidism,
whereby one glycoprotein may stimulate another's receptor.

#23. Thyrotrophinoma
Both a Thyrotrophinoma ('TSHoma') and Thyroid Hormone Resistance
will present with elevated TSH and thyroid hormone levels, however,
the former (TSHoma) is associated with elevated alpha-subunit serum
levels.

#24. a), b) and c) (option e)
POMC is broken down into ACTH, Alpha-Melanocyte stimulating
hormone, beta-endorphin and gamma-melanocyte stimulating
hormone.

<u>#25.</u> c) Primary Gonadal Failure
Primary Gonadal Failure will be associated with increased FSH and LH to attempt to compensate for the hormonal deficiency. In clinical situations such as Turner's, Klinefelter or Prader-Willi Syndrome, hypertrophy of the gonadotrophes may be noted.

<u>#26.</u> c) and d) (option e)
Craniopharyngiomas are suprasellar lesions, and therefore initially compress the optic chiasm from above, forming an inferior bitemporal hemianopia. As pituitary tumours initially compress the optic chiasm from below, the initial abnormality is superior bitemporal hemianopia. In practice, however, this often goes unnoticed by the patient until full bitemporal hemianopia is present.

<u>#27.</u> d) Non-functioning Adenoma
Non-functioning adenomas are the commonest overall pituitary tumour, followed by Prolactinomas.

<u>#28.</u> c) Prolactinomas
Prolactinomas are the second most common pituitary tumour, but the most common 'functional' pituitary tumour overall.

<u>#29.</u> d) Prolactin
Prolactin is under the inhibitory control of dopamine, not a stimulatory hormone. The remaining hormones listed are stimulated by releasing factors.

<u>#30.</u> c) Pineal Gland
The Pineal Gland is responsible for the release of melatonin; the Suprachiasmatic Nucleus of the Hypothalamus controls the circadian rhythm.

<u>#31.</u> c) Parinaud's syndrome
Parinaud's syndrome may result from mid-brain tumours (such as a pinealoma) or infarction, leading to loss of vertical up-gaze, convergence-retraction nystagmus, diplopia, hyporeflexia of the pupils and bilateral lid retraction.

<u>#32.</u> e) Non-functioning adenoma
This case vignette is demonstrative of a non-functioning adenoma. The prolactin is mildly above the reference range, in keeping with

hyperprolactinaemia as a result of pituitary stalk interruption. A macroprolactinoma is much more likely to present with serum prolactin levels above 4,000mU/L. Whilst a microadenoma presents with levels below 4,000mU/L, they are not associated with 'mass effect' or hypopituitarism. The IGF-1 level is decreased in this patient, suggesting the beginning of hypopituitarism from expansion of the macroadenoma. An important caveat to be aware: The 'Hook Effect' occurs due to antigen saturation of the measuring and capturing antibodies, leading to spuriously low prolactin levels – this is repeated in a diluted sample to obtain the true value. Pituitary infarction would present with hypoprolactinaemia (think Sheehan's Syndrome).

#33. a) and b) (option d)
The elevated prolactin inhibits the release of gonadotrophins, which contributes to the reduction in testosterone in this case. Moreover, as the IGF-1 is suppressed, the next trophic hormones to be lost in hypopituitarism are the gonadotrophes, therefore this may be present and further precipitating the testosterone deficiency. Although FSH and LH are within the reference range, this is inappropriately normal in the setting of low testosterone where it should be elevated to attempt to compensate.

#34. a) Pituitary Macroadenoma
This patient had a spuriously low prolactin level with the first measurement due to the 'hook effect', whereby excess antigen over-saturates the antibodies, leading to a falsely depleted level. This is overcome by repeating in a diluted sample. The 'hook effect' may occur when levels are typically greater than 1,000mU/L. It is unlikely that in one week the tumour has significantly increased in size and secretion of prolactin. Macroprolactin is biochemically inactive prolactin that is complexed with antibodies – this is not the case as this patient is symptomatic and has radiological and biochemical confirmation of progressive hypopituitarism.

#35. b) Gonadotrophes
Although non-functional, most non-functional adenomas are histologically traced to gonadotrophes. The hyper-secretion of gonadotrophins, however, is rarely (if ever) seen. Alpha or beta-subunits may occasionally be elevated. Non-functioning adenomas are the commonest overall pituitary tumour.

#36. b) 10%
*Around 10% of the population will harbour a pituitary incidentaloma
on MRI (higher at autopsy), therefore this must always be kept in mind
prior to preforming an MRI for a hyper-secretory disorder (such as
pituitary incidentaloma in hyperthyroidism) leading to an incorrect
diagnosis.*

#37. b) 1cm
*Below 1cm an adenoma is designated as a 'micro'-adenoma, and
above 1cm, designated as a 'macro'-adenoma. Macroadenomas are
more likely to present with the 'mass-effect' and progressive pituitary
insufficiency.*

#38. d) Prolactinoma
*D2 receptors are present within prolactinomas, and Dopamine
Agonists (such as bromocriptine) will drastically shrink prolactinomas
(macro, giant and microprolactinomas), making surgery second (rather
than first) line. All of the other options are best treated with
transsphenoidal surgical resection, with medication only used as
second line/adjunctive therapy.*

#39. a) GH > LH & FSH > TSH> ACTH
*Although the order may vary slightly in textbooks, this is the most
frequent suggestion across medical literature, and the order for which
the author has encountered most frequently. Prolactin levels are rarely
decreased as most cases are a result from an adenoma, leading to
stalk compression and resultant hyperprolactinaemia.*

#40. e) Headache
*There is a very poor correlation between adenoma size and headaches,
and surgery does not always improve the headaches. Stretching of the
diaphragma sellae is the proposed pathophysiology. If
severe/unremitting, then surgery can be considered; moreover, in the
setting of acute, severe headaches, one must consider pituitary
apoplexy (bleeding/infarction of adenoma). Many patients are
managed conservatively, by avoiding headache triggers.*

#41. c) Ki-67
*This is a histological marker of proliferation; above 3% is more likely to
suggest an aggressive mass.*

__#42.__ b) Incidentaloma
The prolactin in this case is unremarkable, with an inappropriate
request for an MRI head and the identification of an incidentaloma.
The lack of libido, headaches and normal biochemical findings are
more likely due to the commencement of sertraline, rather than the
incidentaloma; it is important to note that SSRI medications may
present with minimally increased prolactin (for which once should
withdraw the medication and re-measure if appropriate).

__#43.__ d) Tumour size does not correlate with headache; there is no
guarantee that surgery will improve the headache
There is a very poor correlation between tumour size and headache;
this patient must be made aware that the incidental lesion is very
unlikely to be the cause of the headaches, and the risks of surgery at
the moment outweigh the benefits.

__#44.__ c) Chiari-Frommel occurs in females who have recently given
birth; Ahumada-del Castillo presents without recent delivery
Both conditions present with galactorrhoea and amenorrhoea that is
prolonged in a mother who is not nursing her child; the distinction is
that Chiari-Frommel occurs in those who have recently delivered,
however, Ahumada-del Castillo occurs in those who have not given
birth.

__#45.__ a) SUNCT Headache (Short-lasting, unilateral neuralgiform
headache attacks with conjunctival injection and tearing)
SUNCT Headaches are categorised as a 'Trigeminal Autonomic
Cephalgia' (alongside SUNA, cluster headaches, and paroxysmal
hemicrania). SUNCT (Short-lasting, unilateral neuralgiform headache
attacks with conjunctival injection and tearing) is rarely related to
posterior cranial fossa pathologies or pituitary adenomas. Symptoms
of this disorder include unilateral stabbing/burning periocular pain
autonomic symptomatology such as lacrimation, conjunctival injection,
rhinorrhoea or nasal congestion. The absence of conjunctival injection
or lacrimation suggests SUNA (Short-Lasting Unilateral Neuralgiform
Headache Attacks with Cranial Autonomic Symptoms). The diagnosis
of SUNCT is very rare and may initially be misdiagnosed as Trigeminal
Neuralgia (from cavernous sinus invasion). Trigeminal Autonomic
Cephalgias responds to Indomethicin, however, this is less likely with
SUNCT, which may respond to lidocaine and/or lamotrigine. Removal
of the adenoma may improve symptoms.

#46. a) 10%
Around 10% of microincidentalomas will enlarge to become macroincidentalomas. This is often very reassuring for patients.

#47. a) Knosp Classification System
The Knosp Classification System is used to determine the 'likelihood' of cavernous sinus invasion by a pituitary adenoma. Three lines (medial tangent, intercarotid and lateral tangent) are drawn between the supraclinoid and intracavernous portions of the internal carotid artery on an MRI. The lines are used to grade the invasion:
- o Grade 0: No invasion (medial to medial tangent line)
- o Grade 1: No invasion (between medial tangent & intercarotid line)
- o Grade 2: Invasion possible (between intercarotid & lateral tangent line)
- o Grade 3: Invasion probable
  - ➤ 3A: Above intracavernous ICA into superior cavernous sinus
  - ➤ 3B: Below intracavernous ICA into inferior cavernous sinus
- o Grade 4: Invasion definite (intracavernous ICA completely surrounded)

#48. b) Houssay's Phenomenon
Loss of ACTH and GH due to likely pituitary insufficiency post-resection may improve one's glycaemic status, however, as with this vignette, patients may develop hypoglycaemic episodes.

#49. c) Macroprolactin
This patient demonstrates asymptomatic hyperprolactinaemia. An anterior pituitary hormone panel and an MRI are both unremarkable, for which one should consider a diagnosis of 'macroprolactin', with IgG bound to prolactin molecules (physiologically inert). This can be managed by laboratory technicians mixing polyethylene glycol to the serum which precipitates macroprolactin prior to the immunoassay used.

#50. e) Mandibular Division of the Trigeminal Nerve
*The Mandibular Division of the Trigeminal Nerve does **not** pass through the Cavernous Sinus; the remaining options do.*

#51. c) Frontal Lobe
The frontal lobe is rarely involved in an expanding macroadenoma; classically, this presents with personality change, lack of motivation and anosmia.

#52. a) Prolactin
In 25% of cases, Growth-Hormone secreting adenomas may co-secrete Prolactin. This is most commonly due to a dimorphous adenoma, containing both somaotrophes and lactotrophes. Less commonly, this may be due to the presence of mammosomatotrophes (which produce both Growth Hormone and Prolactin). Very infrequently, this is due to an acidophil stem-cell adenoma, or synchronous Growth-Hormone and Prolactin-secreting adenomas.

#53. f) All of the above
Whilst diabetes insipidus is not always present with hypopituitarism, it is more common with concurrent hypothalamic injury and pituitary stalk compression. A mass within the pituitary gland and diabetes insipidus is (infrequently) associated with pituitary metastases.

#54. b) 30-50%
Up to half of all non-functioning macroadenomas will enlarge over the next ten years (compared to 10% of microadenomas); therefore, surgery is warranted for non-functioning macroadenomas.

#55. c) Parathyroid Adenoma, Pituitary Adenoma, Testicular Carcinoma
Multiple Endocrine Neoplasia Type 4, an extremely uncommon familial condition, presents with parathyroid and pituitary adenomas, in addition to reproductive, renal or adrenal neoplasia.

#56. e) Laron-Type Dwarfism
Laron-Type Dwarfism is an autosomal recessive condition, most common amongst those with semitic ancestry. The disease is caused by mutations in the growth hormone receptor, therefore although GH levels are elevated, IGF-1 is depleted. Moreover, micropenis, craniofacial abnormalities, delayed puberty, hypoglycaemia, disproportional post-natal growth and a hypoplastic nasal bridge are frequently identified.

#57. d) Alcohol inhibits the release of vasopressin from the posterior pituitary gland; Smoking increases the release of vasopressin from the posterior pituitary gland
Both Alcohol and Smoking must therefore be discontinued prior to a water-deprivation test, as they have the potential to interfere with the measurements of urine and plasma osmolality.

<u>#58.</u> c) von-Willebrand Factor
Desmopressin may be used in both the treatment of Haemophilia A and von-Willebrand Disease; stimulation of the V2 receptor results in the release of von-Willebrand Factor from Weibel-Palade bodies within the endothelium. von-Willebrand Factor furthermore carries (and therefore increases levels of) Factor VIII.

<u>#59.</u> d) Smooth muscle contraction
The V1 receptor functions in contraction of smooth muscles, and therefore may increase vascular resistance in states of shock.

<u>#60.</u> b) ACTH
Vasopressin (in addition to supraoptic and paraventricular hypothalamic nuclei) is also produced in the parvocellular nuclei and may travel through the hypophyseal portal circulation to stimulate CRH, with resultant ACTH release.

<u>#61.</u> c) No; Acromegaly can still be present due to the pulsatile release of growth hormone from the pituitary gland.
Due to the pulsatile release of GH, a 'random' level is not used to either diagnose or rule-out acromegaly. IGF-1 represent the 24-hour serum value in relation to the previous day's GH release. With the clinical history and correlation, a single IGF-1 level may be used to diagnose or exclude Acromegaly.

<u>#62.</u> d) Due to the long-half-life of TSH and the low amplitude of pulses, one measurement is satisfactory to assess the underlying thyroid pathology
A single measurement of TSH is satisfactory to determine the thyroid (dys)function. TSH has a long half-life and is released in low pulse amplitudes.

<u>#63.</u> b) Corticosteroids inhibit the release of gonadotrophins
Cushing's Disease is most commonly a result of a microadenoma, and therefore mass effect and direct compression of gonadotrophes is unlikely. Corticosteroids are known to inhibit GnRH, and subsequently decrease gonadotrophin release.

<u>#64.</u> b) Prolactin
Prolactin is elevated post-seizure activity and is occasionally measured to confirm a true seizure over pseudo-seizure.

#65. a) Growth Hormone
Ghrelin directly stimulates the release of Growth Hormone.

#66. e) and f) (option g)
Occasionally microprolactinomas are too small to be visualised on MRI non-contrast. This is referred to as 'idiopathic hyperprolactinaemia'. These will respond to dopamine agonists.

#67. g) All of the above will increase prolactin levels
Prolactin will increase during times of stress (such as venipuncture). Moreover, levels are increased in both renal and liver failure. Occasionally, ectopic production of prolactin will be noted with certain cancers. Pregnancy and PCOS are further states with hyperprolactinaemia (the latter of which is incompletely understood).

#68. d) Pasireotide
Pasireotide is a somatostatin receptor agonist, used in the management of Acromegaly. Prolactinomas are shrunk by Dopamine Agonists. The oral contraceptive pill can be used in patients, however, similar to a prolactinoma, amenorrhoea may occur, and it is not a useful indicator to the degree of hyperprolactinaemia (moreover, it does not shrink the tumour).

#69. c) Quinagolide
Bromocriptine and Cabergoline are considered safe during pregnancy, with bromocriptine being the best studied. Quinagolide is a known teratogen (stillbirth, spontaneous abortion, ectopic pregnancy and congenital malformations) and therefore must not be prescribed in females planning to conceive.

#70. d) The patients are likely to respond to cabergoline
Around 15% of patients 'resistant' to bromocriptine will respond to cabergoline which is more effective. A patient should not be labelled as 'resistant' until all dopamine agonist medications have been trialled.

#71. b) Cabergoline
Cabergoline has the least amount of side effects and may be preferrable to patients as it does not require daily dosing (prescribed twice weekly).

#72. c) Valvular Fibrosis

Cabergoline has the potential to cause valvular fibrosis, and therefore guidelines (although to varying degrees) suggest periodic echocardiogram monitoring. It should be noted that this risk occurs at high dosages when cabergoline is used daily in Parkinson's Disease (>3mg daily for over six months) and is extremely unlikely in the setting of a prolactinoma (twice-weekly, low-dosages). The risk, however, increase when there is partial resistance, requiring an increased dosage of cabergoline.

#73. c) 5-HT$_{2B}$

Cabergoline is an agonist at the 5-HT$_{2B}$ receptor, which is associated with valvular fibrosis at high dosages prescribed (over a chronic period).

#74. a), b) and c) (option e)

Dopamine Agonist Resistance refers to the following:
> o *Failure to normalise prolactin*
> o *Failure to restore fertility in patients receiving standard doses*
> o *Failure to decrease the adenoma to below 50% of its size*

#75. d) Dopamine agonists may be discontinued after two years if normoprolactinaemia is present in addition to the absence of a visible tumour on an MRI

After two years, patients may be considered for discontinuation of the dopamine agonists and are monitored every three months in the first year, followed by annual prolactin measurements (and an MRI if prolactin is raised above the reference range). The risk of recurrence is associated with both the prolactin level and adenoma size at diagnosis. Recurrence is more likely within the first year of withdrawal.

#76. a) Medication to be discontinued, as less than 5% of microadenomas will enlarge during pregnancy (risk of enlargement due to both oestrogen stimulation and withdrawal of medication). Patients to be followed-up in each trimester

Microprolactinomas are very unlikely to enlarge during gestation, and dopamine agonists are best withdrawn at the earliest demonstration of pregnancy. Patients are to be monitored in each trimester, and medications will be recommened if symptomatic growth is evident. Prolactin levels during pregnancy are of little value, as they will naturally be raised. Macroprolactinomas however, may enlarge in up to 30%, and therefore evidence on non-contrast MRI (or symptomatic) of an increase in adenoma size warrants dopamine agonist therapy.

#77. c) and d) (option e)
*Dopamine Agonists inhibit lactation, and therefore in patients with a microprolactinoma that did **not** increase in size during pregnancy, are allowed to breast-feed. There is no risk of pituitary hypertrophy despite the increased prolactin from breast-feeding. In patients who required medication during pregnancy however, it is more important to continue the medication in the post-partum and therefore breast-feeding is not appropriate.*

#78. c) 40-60%
The chance of remission for a microadenoma after pregnancy is between 40-60%.

#79. b) Dopamine Agonist
Dopamine Agonists are always first line in the management of a prolactinoma of any size; should cystic components be present in a macroadenoma (and hence little shrinkage), then surgery is considered (but only after a trial of medication).

#80. e) Pituitary Apoplexy
Neurosurgical evacuation is the treatment of choice for pituitary apoplexy, which is defined as infarction/haemorrhage of the pituitary gland. Pituitary Apoplexy presents as a severe headache, altered level of consciousness, visual impairment and other cranial nerve palsies.

#81. c) Giant Prolactinoma
A Giant (Invasive) Prolactinoma is defined as a tumour greater than four centimetres, with greater than two-centimetre suprasellar extension. Prolactin levels are significantly elevated and risk a falsely lowered level due to the hook effect. Giant Prolactinomas are more prevalent in middle-aged men and may be related to a prior history of radiation. During treatment, there is a heightened risk of pituitary apoplexy, for which patients must be made aware of and closely monitored. As the prolactin is significantly elevated, normoprolactinaemia is not always achievable (and hypogonadism will therefore not always be reversed).

#82. f) All of the above will increase the release of prolactin
Prolactin can be increased by physical stimuli (such as nipple-rings, shingles, suckling, breast examination) and hypothyroidism (from increased TSH and TRH).

#83. d) Risperidone
Risperidone is notorious for to severe hyperprolactinaemia; other atypical antipsychotics are less likely to lead to hyperprolactinaemia (more common with typical antipsychotics). Risperidone accumulates within the pituitary gland as it poorly penetrates the blood-brain barrier.

#84. h) All of the above
All of the options listed may be attempted; it is important to note which antipsychotic the patient was started on, as some may demonstrate transient (versus chronic) hyperprolactinaemia. Aripiprazole is a novel agonist/antagonist and has not been demonstrated to worsen psychotic features when combined with other antipsychotics for the management of antipsychotic-induced hyperprolactinaemia.

#85. c) Thyroid-Receptor Beta-2
Beta-2 thyroid receptors are present within the anterior pituitary, for which mutations can lead to Refetoff syndrome (resistance to thyroid hormone). Beta-1 is expressed in the liver and kidney. Alpha-1 is expressed throughout multiple tissues, including cardiac muscle, skeletal muscle and the central nervous system. Notably, although present in various tissues, alpha-2 is unable to bind to Triiodothyronine.

#86. b) and c) (option d)
Chronic corticosteroid administration depletes the release of Growth Hormone and inhibits GnRH(and subsequently gonadotrophin release). Acute administration of corticosteroids, however, may increase Growth Hormone release (as part of the stress response).

#87. a) and d) (option f)
Factors which predict the risk of developing hyperprolactinaemia include
> *o Female*
> *o Adolescence/reproductive age*

o Parity
o D2 receptor mutation (4x risk with TaqIA Aq and A0241G)
o Increased dosage
o Typical antipsychotic

#88. c) Chiari-Frommel Syndrome
*Chiari-Frommel Syndrome, which occurs for greater than six months, presents with galactorrhoea, amenorrhoea and prolonged anovulation in non-breastfeeding mothers. Resolution may occur. The cause is incompletely understood. Ahumada-del Castillo Syndrome presents similarly, but in females who have **not** recently given birth. Forbes-Albright Syndrome occurs similarly, but with a pituitary tumour and without childbirth or nursing.*

#89. c) and d) (option g)
Familial tumours (such as a macroprolactinoma) are more likely to be aggressive, hyperfunctional and less responsive to treatment.

#90. a) Temozolomide
Despite the rarity of a pituitary carcinoma, an initial response followed by an absent response to a dopamine agonist is suggestive of a pituitary carcinoma. Temozolomide is a promising treatment (alkylating chemotherapeutic agent).

#91. a) and b) (option e)
The Gs pathway is involved in the secretion of thyroid hormones (as well as glandular growth/differentiation, and iodide uptake), whereas the Gq pathway stimulates the rate-limiting step of hormone synthesis (iodide organification).

#92. c) Saturation of 11-Beta-Hydroxysteroid Dehydrogenase Type 2
11-Beta-Hydroxysteroid Dehydrogenase Type 2, located near mineralocorticoid receptors (dominant within the kidney), function to inactivate cortisol into cortisone. With ectopic ACTH Syndrome, there is excessive release of ACTH (and therefore cortisol), with the enzyme becoming 'saturated' leading to pronounced mineralocorticoid effects such as hypokalaemia.

#93. c) Testosterone is converted to oestrogen through the aromatase enzyme, which may increase the release of prolactin

Although very infrequently, case reports have depicted a paradoxical rise in prolactin after administering testosterone, due to the peripheral conversion into oestrogens. Guidance is limited; however, some clinicians recommend aromatase enzyme inhibitors to be prescribed alongside the testosterone replacement.

#94. a) Prolactin

Whilst the mechanism is largely unknown, limited evidence has suggested prolactin is furthermore important in the production of foetal surfactant.

#95. e) All of the above are correct

All of the listed options are known to occur with prolactin.

#96. b) Oxytocin

Oxytocin, released from the posterior pituitary gland, functions alongside prolactin during breast-feeding, whereby suckling promotes the let-down of milk (oxytocin) and lactation (prolactin).

#97. a) CTLA-4 Immunotherapy

CTLA-4 Immunotherapy, most commonly ipilimumab, may lead hypophysitis (in addition to various other endocrine manifestations, such as adrenal insufficiency, diabetes mellitus and thyroid dysfunction).

#98. c) and d) (option e)

Secondary hypothyroidism presents differently to primary hypothyroidism; there is likely to be other anterior pituitary hormone deficiencies, and therefore instead of classic symptoms such as weight gain, with concurrent ACTH deficiency weight loss may be noted. Similarly, instead of cold intolerance, 'hot flushes' may be demonstrated due to hypogonadotrophic hypogonadism. Goitres are not typically seen, as there is a lack of TSH and its resultant trophic effects.

#99. c) Vitamin B6 (Pyridoxine)

Both a deficiency of this vitamin, as well as toxicity results in neuropathy. Moreover, Vitamin B6 is known to inhibit the release of

prolactin in laboratory studies; the effect of this within humans is less clear.

#100. d) Vasoactive Intestinal Peptide (VIP)
As a result, prolactin measurements are taken after an overnight fast, as recent ingestion may alter the results.

#101. b) Copeptin
Copeptin is released alongside vasopressin and Neurophysin (common precursor). Copeptin has been noted to have a mild stimulatory effect upon prolactin release.

#102. e) GH and Prolactin
The remaining options act through a G-protein receptor (with secondary chemical messenger). GH and Prolactin act through the JAK-STAT pathway.

#103. c) Tyrosine Hydroxylase
Tyrosine hydroxylase is the rate-limiting step in the synthesis of catecholamines and dopamine and is upregulated in hyperprolactinaemia. This functions to decrease prolactin.

#104. d) Rapid Eye Movement (REM) Sleep
Prolactin is elevated during REM Sleep; literature suggests that prolactin may actually modulate the transition into REM sleep.

#105. b) Vitamin C
Ascorbate (Vitamin C) is required for the final hydrolysis, resulting in the release of Oxytocin.

#106. b) Cholecystokinin
Oxytocin levels are noted to be increased following gastric distention; in-vivo studies have demonstrated this to be a likely response to Cholecystokinin (CCK).

#107. b) Oxytocin
Due to the similarities between vasopressin and oxytocin, excessive oxytocin (such as that used for labour), may lead to an ADH-response, with hyponatraemia.

#108. c) and e) (option g)
*SIADH must be differentiated from Cerebral Salt-Wasting (CSW), due
to the differing managements. Both may occur post-subarachnoid
haemorrhage, however, SIADH is much more likely. SIADH is a result of
inappropriate water retention (ADH release) and presents with
euvolaemia, whereas CSW is a result of inappropriate salt-wasting (in
the urine), and there presents with hypovolaemia. The treatment of
SIADH is fluid restriction, whereas saline must be administered in
cerebral salt wasting syndrome. Laboratory tests are poor to
distinguish between the two entities as both will present with
hyponatraemia, increased urine osmolality, increased urine sodium
and decreased serum uric acid; therefore, CSW heavily relies upon
physical signs of hypovolaemia.*

#109. e) Acromegaly
*The great majority (~95%) of cases of Acromegaly are a result of a
pituitary **macro**adenoma. Less frequent causes include hypothalamic
masses leading to GHRH hyper-secretion, ectopic IGF-1 or GHRH
paraneoplastic syndrome*

#110. c) MRI with contrast with 2mm slices
*This is the standard modality for identifying acromegaly
(macroadenomas).*

#111. e) Gigantism
*Gigantism occurs prior to growth plate closure (due to increased GH
such as a macroadenoma), whereas Acromegaly occurs in adults, once
the growth plates have closed.*

#112. b) Prolactin
*Prolactin is co-secreted with GH in 30% of cases of Acromegaly and is a
cause of hyperprolactinaemia in Acromegaly apart from pituitary stalk
compression. This may be due to mammosomatotroph cells within the
adenoma (Releasing both GH and prolactin), mixed adenomas
(bimorphous; with both somatotrophes and lactotrophes), or less
commonly, stem-cell (acidophilic) adenomas.*

#113. b) Five to Ten Years
*Acromegaly is frequently delayed in diagnosis, due to the non-specific
complaints. On average, it takes around seven years until a diagnosis is
delivered.*

#114. e) 95%
~95% of cases of Acromegaly are a result of a pituitary adenoma – acromegaly is more likely to be a result of a macroadenoma and therefore visual complaints are a common feature compared to Cushing's Disease, which is more frequently a microadenoma (and therefore no visual impairment).

#115. d) All of the above
All of the dietary options listed (excessive dairy products, glucose and protein) are known to interfere with (and potentially raise) IGF-1 measurements.

#116. d) Cannot be determined at eight weeks postoperatively
*Although elevated levels of IGF-1 and GH post-operatively are highly convincing for inadequate tumour resection, one must remember these will be elevated as part of the stress response. Most authors suggest waiting **at least twelve weeks** prior to post-operative measurement of IGF-1 and GH due to the long half-life of IGF-1 (of up to three months). An MRI should also be delayed, to allow involution of gel foam and the fat packing.*

#117. d) Pituitary Adenoma (Empty Sella Syndrome)
Whilst the MRI report suggests 'limited pituitary tissue, the full description is quite suggestive of Empty Sella Syndrome. In this patient, the sella turcica is defective and is filled (partially or completely) with cerebrospinal fluid, with a compressed/flattened pituitary gland. Most patients are asymptomatic; however, deficiencies may occur with compression. Interestingly, hyper-secretory states (and adenomas) within the 'flattened' pituitary gland have been demonstrated (empty sella on MRI may hinder the correct diagnosis and lead to unnecessary explorations for ectopic GHRH-producing neoplasms).

#118. d) Oral Oestrogen
Oral (not transdermal) oestrogen demonstrates a first-pass effect with the inhibition of Growth Hormone upon the liver; IGF-1 levels are lower on oral oestrogen and higher dosages of GH replacement are required.

#119. d) IGF-1 levels decrease; GH levels decrease
It is very important that IGF-1 levels are interpreted with the patient's age in mind, as Growth Hormone secretion decreases with age, and

therefore the levels of IGF-1 decrease (highest during puberty and pregnancy).

#120. c) 1.0ng/mL
Although the proposed 'cut-off' is 0.4ng/mL, many assays cannot detect such low levels of Growth Hormone, and therefore levels above 1.0ng/mL are considered diagnostic for acromegaly.

#121. f) All of the above
All the options listed can lead to depleted IGF-levels; for this reason, the interpretation of IGF-1 must always be done with the full clinical history. It may be more important to treat the comorbidities and then measure IGF-1 once stabilised.

#122. b) Hypophosphataemia
Hyperphosphataemia may be present in up to 70% of patients with acromegaly, hypothesised to be a result of IGF-1 acting upon tubular cells to reabsorb phosphate. Moreover, hypercalcaemia (and hypercalciuria) may be present, as well as hypertriglyceridaemia and hyperglycaemia.

#123. e) All of the above
Acromegaly increases the risk of colorectal cancer, for which increased colon screening is mandatory. Moreover, multinodular goitre formation (thyroid) can also occur, again, with an increased risk of cancer for which sonographic assessment is mandated. Also less commonly discussed, medical literature suggests a potentially increased prevalence of melanoma, stomach, uterine and oesophageal cancers with acromegaly.

#124. d) Cardiovascular Disease
Whilst all the options listed contribute to increased morbidity, the mortality is most often a result of cardiovascular disease (such as hypertension).

#125. a) and b) (option e)
'Active Symptoms' are an important concept; many of the phenotypical manifestations of Acromegaly such as increased shoe size, diastema, prognathism et cetera will be permanent, and do not reliably help to distinguish active versus inactive disease. Sweating and hypertension are two common 'active symptoms'.

<u>#126.</u> a), b) and c) (option g)
Diabetes and Hyperhidrosis are unlikely to continue and will improve after treatment. In contrast, sleep apnoea, arthralgia and valvulopathy represent tissue disturbance/damage, for which it will not progress, but may not improve.

<u>#127.</u> e) All of the above may cause false positives
Chronic impairment of the liver and kidneys, as well as adolescence, malnutrition and diabetes mellitus may lead to a false positive result. Additionally, chronic opiate administration (addiction) has been noted to cause a false-positive result.

<u>#128.</u> b) Diabetes Mellitus
A paradoxical increase in GH may be noted in up to 1/3 of patients after the oral glucose tolerance test; this is most likely due to diabetes mellitus.

<u>#129.</u> c) Maxillofacial Reconstruction
Maxillofacial Reconstruction should be considered once post-operative results demonstrate successful resection; this is recommended as the deformities caused by acromegaly are likely to be permanent.

<u>#130.</u> c) and d) (option g)
*By no means does this mean that the surgery was a 'failure'. Debulking a macroadenoma will result in heightened sensitivity to treatment (such as with somatostatin receptor analogues). The majority of Acromegaly cases are due to a **macro**adenoma, for which extension is more likely, coupling to a decreased likelihood for complete resection.*

<u>#131.</u> d) One Year
Patients should be counselled that it can take up to one year for improvement in visual deficits post-transsphenoidal surgical resection.

<u>#132.</u> d) Surgery
Surgery is first line for Acromegaly, regardless of the location of the tumour (i.e., pituitary macroadenoma or ectopic paraneoplastic syndrome).

<u>#133.</u> a) Gallstones
Somatostatin receptor analogues are associated with an increased risk of gallstone formation; this is due to somatostatin inhibiting the

contraction of the gallbladder. Asymptomatic gallstones are found in up to half of all patients within the first two years of treatment with this class of medication, however, sonogram is not warranted unless symptomatic. Moreover, somatostatin receptor analogues are associated with an improvement in headaches. This class of medication may cause bradycardia, constipation and hair loss. Hypoglycaemia is not an adverse effect of this medication.

#134. a) Pasireotide
Whilst somatostatin analogues may later the glycaemic index, the risk of worsened hyperglycaemia is far greater with pasireotide.

#135. d) Somatostatin Receptor Ligands normalise IGF-1 levels in up to 60% and reduce tumour size in ~50%. Pegvisomant decreases IGF-1 levels in around 90% but may increase tumour size.
*It is imperative to note that Pegvisomant can increase the tumour size in up to 5% of patients and should therefore never be prescribed if the tumour is close to or abutting the optic chiasm. Serial MRI scans of the pituitary are therefore mandatory. Patients are also at risk for elevated liver function tests and injection site reactions. Growth hormone levels will inevitably be elevated as Pegvisomant functions as a receptor antagonist, and therefore should **not** be measured in these patients.*

#136. a) Turner's Syndrome
Turner's Syndrome patients are occasionally treated with Growth Hormone injections to increase their height; close follow-up is required to prevent 'iatrogenic acromegaly'.

#137. d) Densely Granulated (more responsive to somatostatin receptor ligands); Sparsely Granulated (less responsive to somatostatin receptor ligands)
Densely Granulated Tumours are smaller in size, however, are more biochemically active (and hence more responsive to medication). Sparsely Granulated Tumours, however, are more likely in younger patients, and are more 'aggressive' compared to Densely Granulated Tumours (therefore less responsive to medication).

#138. d) Infrequent, but expected side-effect of the medication
This patient is likely taking Pegvisomant injections, which increase the serum GH level (GH should not be measured in these patients). Moreover, the adenoma may increase in size on this medication, and

as in this vignette, has reached the optic chiasm, requiring immediate termination of Pegvisomant. Recurrence of disease does not fit with the clinical history.

#139. a), b), c) and d) (option g)
All of the options listed are potential side-effects of Pegvisomant Injection.

#140. e) All of the above
Stereotactic radiosurgery requires a single appointment (instead of multiple), and therefore is more preferable for patients as it has a shorter duration of treatment. Moreover, there is a shorter time to remission with stereotactic radiosurgery. Although to varying results, primitive evidence does suggest there may be a decreased risk of cognitive decline and hypopituitarism compared to conventional therapy. It should be noted however, that stereotactic radiosurgery is not appropriate with the mass near the optic chiasm.

#141. c) 50%
At ten years post-radiotherapy, half of all patients will demonstrate hypopituitarism.

#142. b) Acrochordons
Skin tags (also known as Acrochordons, Fibroepithelial Polyps or Papillomas) are present in states of insulin resistance and/or dyslipidaemia, such as Cushing's syndrome, diabetes mellitus, pregnancy and acromegaly. More commonly however, they arise in areas of tight clothing, suggesting a response to chronic irritation.

#143. f) All of the above
Octreotide scanning has many fallacies (as do many endocrine imaging modalities); false-positives can be seen with non-neuroendocrine tumours (such as breast cancer, follicular thyroid adenomas, brain tumours and lymphoma). Moreover, inflammatory conditions such as granulomatous disorders, fibrosis and radiation result in further false positives. Irregular anatomy (such as an accessory spleen) may be misinterpreted as a neuroendocrine tumour.

#144. c) Bronchial Carcinoid
Bronchial Carcinoids are the most common source of ectopic Acromegaly, with the hypersecretion of Growth-Hormone Releasing

Hormone. It should be noted however, that although biochemical acromegaly may be noted with this tumour, the phenotypical presentation is less common (but still possible).

#145. a) Acromegaloidism
This vignette is highly suggestive of Acromegaloidism, which presents with phenotypical acromegaly, however with normal biochemical panels (IGF-1 and GH). Pachydermoperiostosis is characterised by clubbing, skin thickening and hyperhidrosis, and is a classic differential to Acromegaly.

#146. b) Growth Factor
Acromegaloidism is believed to occur due to increased levels of local growth factors.

#147. c) Residual tissue near the optic chiasm
Despite its many advantages over conventional radiotherapy, it is inappropriate to use stereotactic radiotherapy with residual tissue near the optic chiasm.

#148. b) Burned Out Acromegaly
'Burned Out Acromegaly' occurs as a result of self-infarction of an adenoma as a result of increased adenoma size. This leads to 'subclinical pituitary apoplexy', and infarction will therefore lead to an auto-hypophysectomy (preventing hyper-secretion of Growth Hormone). The phenotypical manifestations of acromegaly therefore remain static, and biochemistry may indicate no active disease/normal values.

#149. f) All of the above
Pseudoacromegaly refers to a phenotype similar to acromegaly. This has been described with chronic phenytoin and minoxidil administration, as well as severe, untreated hypothyroidism. Moreover, Type A Insulin Resistance and Ascher's Syndrome are classic causes of pseudoacromegaly.

#150. b) Paget's Disease
Paget's Disease, also known as Osteitis Deformans, can present similarly to Acromegaly, with the classic complaint of hearing loss (from neural compression). Elevated Alkaline Phosphatase and normal calcium (unless immobile) are classic.

#151. b), c) and d) (option f)
Although classically used to confirm GH deficiency, the insulin stress test is used to assess for hypoadrenalism. Prolactin levels may also be measured, as they are released in insulin-induced hypoglycaemic states (increase alongside cortisol and may alleviate the anti-inflammatory effects of glucocorticoids; may also be part of the stress response).

#152. b) Growth Hormone Deficiency
A serum GH (peak) under 5 micrograms/L at any time during hypoglycaemia suggests adult growth-hormone deficiency. The cortisol response is adequate (peak level 600nmol/L).

#153. i) All of the above are contraindications
All of the listed options are contraindications to performing this procedure.

#154. b) and d) (option f)
Severe (untreated) hypothyroidism will impair the released of both growth hormone and cortisol and should be treated prior to the performance of the test for adequate interpretation of results.

#155. b) Cannot be interpreted
Whilst the vignette is attempting to make you select Growth Hormone deficiency (from his previous radiation), as hypoglycaemia is not induced (<2.2mmol/L), Growth Hormone reserve cannot be interpreted. Hypoglycaemia must be induced (under 2.2mmol/L) to adequately assess the GH reserve.

#156. e) 5 micrograms/L
Failure to reach above 5 micrograms/L suggests adult growth hormone deficiency.

#157. d) All of the above
Macimorelin, Glucagon and Arginine-GHRH stimulation tests are also available to assess for Growth Hormone Deficiency, however, Insulin Tolerance Test is considered the gold standard.

#158. e) Six weeks; falsely increases cortisol levels
Cortisol assays involve the measurement of both 'total' and 'free' cortisol; oestrogen is known to increase hepatic synthesis of

corticosteroid binding globulin (CBG), and a resultant increase in
protein-bound cortisol (leading to increased total cortisol). For this
reason, it must be stopped six weeks before the assay is to be
performed.

#159. b) TSH/Free T4
*Levels of T4 may decrease upon Growth Hormone administration (and
may unmask central hypothyroidism).*

#160. h) All of the above are potential complications
*In essence, administration of growth hormone may lead to iatrogenic
acromegaly, with arthralgia, sleep apnoea, myalgia and oedema more
likely than the other options listed.*

#161. a) Obesity
*Obese patients may require an increased dosage of Growth Hormone
as well as oral (but transdermal) oestrogen (premenopausal women
are likely to require a higher dose than postmenopausal women).
Laron-Type Dwarfism is due to GH receptor insensitivity to GH, and
therefore Growth Hormone replacement is not effective. Growth
Hormone is contraindicated in pregnancy and lactation.*

#162. h) Under 18 years of age
*Growth Hormone is occasionally supplied in children with short-stature
for conditions such as Turner's Syndrome; it is not contraindicated in
children.*

#163. d) Creutzfeldt-Jakob Disease
*Creutzfeldt-Jakob Disease was previously transmissible through
cadaveric growth hormone, however, nowadays growth hormone is
synthetic, and this is no longer a concern.*

#164. d) Decreased Insulin Resistance
*Growth Hormone is a diabetogenic hormone, and acromegaly (states
of GH excess) leads to hyperglycaemia and insulin resistance.*

#165. d) GH Response below 3.0micrograms/L (ITT)
*National Institute for Health and Care Excellence (NICE) recommend
the initiation of Growth Hormone if three core criteria are applicable:*
  (1) Peak GH below 3micrograms/L (Insulin Tolerance Test)

(2)   Already replacing other anterior pituitary hormone deficiencies

(3)   Score of at least 11 with the QoL-AGHDA

#166. c) Concentration and Libido
*This is not a category of the questionnaire (although is likely to improve!) – however, concentration and **memory** is. The other options are categories assessed with the questionnaire.*

#167. b) Stalk Compression
Acromegaly is more commonly due to a macroadenoma, for which the mass effect (expansion) and pituitary stalk compression are likely results. The prolactin would be much higher in the case of a prolactinoma (or co-secretion with Growth Hormone). This is unlikely to be due to macroprolactin as there is a demonstrative hypersecretion syndrome present.

#168. d) Urinary Beta-hCG
Amenorrhoea and hyperprolactinaemia are concerning for pregnancy; it is mandatory to rule out pregnancy prior to assessing for a prolactinoma.

#169. c) Repeat Insulin-Stress Test; unlikely to require Growth Hormone by adulthood
The great majority of children (up to 70%) with a case of isolated GH deficiency will have normal results when retested as adults, and therefore this should be assessed within the transition period. It is unlikely it will need to be continued into adulthood.

#170. b) Langerhans Cell Histiocytosis
This case vignette demonstrates the classic triad of Letterer-Siwe Disease (form of Langerhans Cell Histiocytosis): Proptosis, Diabetes Insipidus and osteolytic lesions. Classically, a histology report will comment upon 'Birbeck Granules'.

#171. f) Citalopram
Citalopram presents with SIADH, not nephrogenic diabetes insipidus.

<u>#172.</u> b) and c) (option f)
Amphotericin B may lead to hypomagnesaemia and hypokalaemia (hypomagnesaemia can worsen hypokalaemia). Hypokalaemia is a cause of nephrogenic diabetes insipidus.

<u>#173.</u> c) NSAIDs
NSAIDs enhance the actions of ADH and must be stopped prior to a water deprivation test. The remaining options may interfere with the test, but do not potentiate ADH.

<u>#174.</u> c) Psychogenic Polydipsia
At the start of the test there is dilute urine and hyponatraemia; this patient demonstrates increasing concentration of urine and slightly increasing plasma osmolality with water deprivation, suggestive of psychogenic polydipsia. There is no need to perform the second portion of the test (vasopressin administration).

<u>#175.</u> a) and d)
Both Tolvaptan (ADH antagonist) and Demeclocycline (tetracycline antibiotic) lead to a form of drug-induced nephrogenic diabetes insipidus. Whilst mannitol increases diuresis, it is not appropriate to prescribe this for SIADH. Moreover, a side-effect of Lithium is nephrogenic diabetes insipidus, however it is inappropriate to prescribe for this effect.

<u>#176.</u> d) Lesion within the hypothalamus, heightened thirst sensation
Dipsogenic Diabetes Insipidus may be identified in cases previously considered to be 'psychogenic polydipsia'; this is due to a lesion within the hypothalamus, for which the sensation of thirst is heightened, not decreased, leading to a compelling desire to quench ones' thirst.

<u>#177.</u> b) and c) (option e)
Psychogenic Polydipsia is best differentiated from true diabetes insipidus by:
- *Waking up at night to drink water (rather than urinate)*
- *Daytime urination (no nocturia)*
- *Associated psychiatric disorder*

<u>#178.</u> d) Vasopressin antagonist at V2 receptor
Tolvaptan may be used in the management of SIADH, however the resultant effect will be drug-induced nephrogenic diabetes insipidus.

#179. b) Nephrogenic Diabetes Insipidus
Increased plasma osmolality with relative urinary dilution is present; after administration of vasopressin, the urine osmolality remains diluted, suggestive of nephrogenic diabetes insipidus. A partial response would be expected in partial nephrogenic diabetes insipidus.

#180. c) Cranial Diabetes Insipidus
This would suggest cranial diabetes insipidus; partial cranial diabetes insipidus would be more likely in the setting of recent head injury, and would present with increased urine osmolality, but not above 800mOsm/Kg.

#181. c) MDMA
MDMA (ecstasy) is a common drug of abuse amongst adolescents, which can lead to severe thirst. Patients may drink several litres of water following ingestion and will present with hyponatraemia as the water intake exceeds the kidney's capacity to excrete water, leading to water retention and hyponatraemia.

#182. b) Anticholinergics
Anticholinergic medications (or medications which have anti-cholinergic effects such amitriptyline) present with a dry mouth and can be cause of primary polydipsia.

#183. b) Carbamazepine
This case vignette is very classic for Trigeminal Neuralgia sequelae; Carbamazepine is used in the management of this disorder, however, may cause SIADH (with orthostatic hypotension, lethargy, hyponatraemia, increased urine osmolality and increased urine sodium).

#184. a) Sickle Cell Trait
Whilst carriers are asymptomatic, a peculiar notion may be noted: isothenuria (the inability to concentrate urine).

#185. c) The bright spot is retained in primary polydipsia and nephrogenic diabetes insipidus, but absent in cranial diabetes insipidus
This is a classic exam question! The bright spot can be used to differentiate primary polydipsia from cranial diabetes insipidus

(however, it may be present in nephrogenic diabetes insipidus and should not be used to distinguish from primary polydipsia).

#186. Hyperparathyroidism; Nephrogenic Diabetes Insipidus
This patient has suffered from both an insulinoma and a prolactinoma – it is very likely she has Multiple Endocrine Neoplasia Syndrome Type I, which would also predispose to hyperparathyroidism. Her current presentation is suggestive of hypercalcaemia (and resultant nephrogenic diabetes insipidus).

#187. a), b) and c) (option e)
All of the options listed are reasons to terminate the water deprivation test.

#188. d) Placenta; Gestational Diabetes Insipidus
A rare cause of diabetes insipidus may occur during pregnancy, whereby the placenta releases 'vasopressinase' which metabolises vasopressin. This may result in Gestational Diabetes Insipidus, however, the clinical relevance of this is debatable.

#189. c) Results are indistinguishable from nephrogenic diabetes insipidus
Chronic water ingestion in excessive amounts may lead to downregulation of ADH release and receptors within the kidney. The resultant medullary gradient is altered. When a water-deprivation test is performed, polyuria persists as the gradient may be insufficient to reabsorb water (similar to nephrogenic diabetes insipidus).

#190. c) Hyponatraemia and decreased renal excretion of free water (serum dilution) in patients drinking excess alcohol and poor dietary intake
Beer Potomania will be seen in chronic alcoholics; as stated, it presents with hyponatraemia from decreased water excretion from poor solute formation (leading to increased reabsorption of water). This is coupled with a poor dietary intake.

#191. d) Autosomal Dominant Inheritance
Wolfram Syndrome is an autosomal recessive (not dominant) disorder characterised by a mutation in the WFS1 Gene. The condition is also referred to as DIDMOAD, as this represents the acronym of the clinical findings:

- *Diabetes Insipidus*
- *Diabetes Mellitus*
- *Optic Atrophy*
- *Deafness*

#192. d) Females develop pituitary apoplexy twice as often as males
All of the listed options are correct apart from option d). For reasons that are unknown, males develop pituitary apoplexy nearly twice as often as females.

#193. a) Non-functioning adenoma
Pituitary apoplexy is most likely with a non-functioning macroadenoma; prolactinomas are the most common cause of subclinical pituitary apoplexy.

#194. d) All of the above are correct
All the options listed are correct; subclinical pituitary apoplexy may occasionally be beneficial as it leads to an autohypophysectomy of a hypersecreting adenoma. Prolactinomas are the commonest underlying tumour in such a case, and it is more likely to occur in females.

#195. b) Hypothalamo-pituitary-adrenal axis
ACTH Deficiency may occur and is life-threatening; therefore, this must be measured and corrected to prevent fatality.

#196. Kallmann's Syndrome
This patient presents with hypogonadotrophic hypogonadism, anosmia and bimanual synkinesis, characteristic for Kallmann's Syndrome. Congenital Isolated Hypogonadotrophic Hypogonadism is the diagnosis when there is no underlying causation identified.

#197. e) Exogenous steroid administration
Exogenous corticosteroid administration must be considered in 'body builders', especially when low testosterone is present. Moreover, a track mark is noted in the antecubital fossa, and he has 'shrunken' testicles, all due to exogenous steroid abuse.

#198. d) Its presence refers to an inactive form conjugated to antibodies, being physiologically inert
Macroprolactin must always be considered in a patient with hyperprolactinaemia who is asymptomatic. Macroprolactin can be 'precipitated' in the serum with polyethylene glycol pre-treatment to avoid an incorrect diagnosis.

#199. a) Cyclic Cushing's Disease
Cyclic Cushing's Disease is a rare manifestation with episodic (cyclical) hypercortisolism; this is best assessed for with urinary free cortisol or late-night salivary cortisol rather than a dexamethasone suppression test.

#200. c) Adrenal Adenoma
Whilst it is extremely unlikely for patients with Cushing's syndrome to become pregnant (as most experience amenorrhoea or oligomenorrhoea), in those who do become pregnant, the most common underlying cause is an adrenal adenoma (rather than a pituitary adenoma).

#201. c) Small-Cell Lung Carcinoma
This presentation is suggestive of ectopic ACTH Syndrome, characterised by an elderly male with a smoking history. Moreover, hypokalaeamia, hyperpigmentation and lack of suppression with the high dose dexamethasone suppression test are key findings. The chest x-ray should be compared to prior images before concluding this is a new mass however, as it could be an incidental, chronic lesion previously identified.

#202. c) Bronchial Carcinoid
Up to 10% of bronchial carcinoids may become suppressed with a high-dose dexamethasone suppression test, which can lead to confusion in the diagnosis.

#203. d) Corticosteroids directly inhibit the responsiveness of GnRH, contributing to inhibition of the release of gonadotrophins
Although it was previously assumed that the hyperandrogenaemia results in decreased FSH and LH release, it is now known that this is not the case. Corticosteroids directly inhibit the responsiveness of GnRH, which result in decreased gonadotrophins. There does not seem to be a strong relationship between androgen levels and amenorrhoea.

#204. e) Pioglitazone
Pioglitazone is an inducer of this enzymatic complex, which would increase the metabolism of dexamethasone. The other options listed are enzyme inhibitors.

#205. e) All of the above
Bacteriuria will metabolise cortisol leading to a false negative. Large amounts of free water ingested prior to the test will increase the filtration and result in false positive results. Creatinine clearance below 60mL/min will decrease proper filtration and therefore falsely low levels in the urine appear. Finally, urinary free cortisol is not sensitive for mild disease, as the urinary measurement measures purely free cortisol and not the corticosteroid metabolites (which are likely to be increased first in mild disease).

#206. a) Hydrochlorothiazide
Hydrochlorothiazide (and occasionally amiloride) are prescribed in nephrogenic diabetes insipidus, as it leads to a paradoxical anti-diuretic effect (from mild hypovolaemia) with resorption of water and sodium.

#207. b) GH deficiency
Septo-optic dysplasia (de Morsier Syndrome) is an uncommon disorder, however, it is important to know that whilst any endocrine deficiency can occur, growth hormone is most commonly deficient.

#208. f) All of the above
All of the listed options interfere with the midnight salivary cortisol measurement. Night-shift workers have an altered circadian rhythm (such as jetlag), for which levels may be elevated. Bovine hormones within dairy products may cross-react with anticortisol antibodies. Smoking/licorice ingestion inhibit 11-beta-hydroxysteroid dehydrogenase type 2 within the salivary glands, preventing the inactivation of cortisol to cortisone. Moreover, sugar or acid-containing foods are known to interfere with the pH of the assay. Hot drink/brushing teeth may cause bleeding for which falsely elevated levels have been documented.

#209. b) Ferritin and iron saturation
Always consider haemochromatosis as a cause of hyperpigmentation/bronze appearance, especially in the setting of

diabetes and hypogonadism. The next most appropriate test would be the ferritin and iron saturation measurements.

#210. b) Dexamethasone-CRH Test
Pseudocushing's can be notoriously difficult to distinguish from cushing's syndrome to the untrained professional. It is helpful to know that skin manifestations (such as proximal muscular atrophy, easy bruising, thinning of the skin) are very unlikely with pseudocushing's disease. The Dexamethasone-CRH Test can be used to distinguish between the two entities, as normal suppression of cortisol will be observed in pseudocushing's but not in cushing's disease.

About the Author

Dr. Barnett is a graduate of the University of Buckingham Medical School (Hons.). His areas of interest include Endocrinology, Diabetes Mellitus, Metabolic Medicine and Chemical Pathology. He is currently enrolled in a 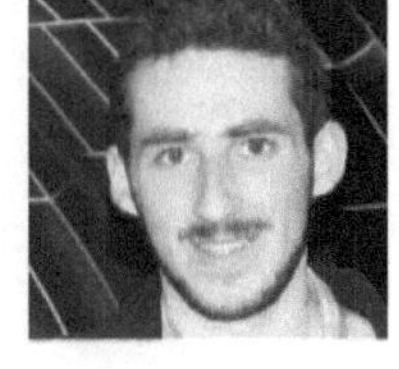 master's in endocrinology at the University of South Wales, in addition to diabetes care at the University of Warwick. Throughout his journey in medicine, he has developed a love for teaching fellow doctors and medical students and hopes to become a professor in Endocrinology and Diabetes, with the privilege of teaching all healthcare professionals.

Dr. Barnett is qualified in the United States of America, the United Kingdom and the State of Israel.

Upcoming Releases:

- Endocrinology Volume II: Reproductive Endocrinology; Parathyroid, Calcium & Bone; and Neuro-Endocrine Tumours.

- Diabetes Revision

- Metabolic Medicine & Clinical Chemistry